The
Iodine
Balancing
Handbook

Optimize Your **DIET,** Regulate **THYROID HORMONES,** and Transform Your **TOTAL-BODY HEALTH**

Malini Ghoshal, RPh, MS

ULYSSES PRESS

Published by:
ULYSSES PRESS
PO Box 3440
Berkeley, CA 94703
www.ulyssespress.com

ISBN: 978-1-64604-453-5
Library of Congress Control Number: 2022944063

Printed in the United States
10 9 8 7 6 5 4 3 2 1

Acquisitions editor: Shelona Belfon
Managing editor: Claire Chun
Editor: Scott Calamar
Proofreader: Kathy Kaiser
Front cover design: Ashley Prine
Interior design and layout: Winnie Liu
Cover artwork: food © Minur/shutterstock.com; scale © Cinderella Design/ shutterstock.com
Interior artwork: page 11 © LuYago/shutterstock.com; page 15 © art4stock/ shutterstock.com; page 16 © Designua/shutterstock.com; pages 95–97 © PegasuStudio/shutterstock.com

This book is dedicated to my mother, Minati Banerjee.
Ma, thank you for always being so caring and supportive.

This book is also dedicated in loving memory
to my father, Asim Kumar Banerjee.
Ba, thank you for teaching me the values of
integrity, ethics, and hard work.

Contents

Note from the Author

The material contained in this book is for informational purposes only. It is not intended to diagnose or treat any health conditions. It should not be interpreted as medical advice. Any errors or omissions are unintentional.

If you have questions about your health, including iodine deficiency or excess, consult with an experienced clinician or an endocrinologist to learn more.

Conditions, symptoms, diagnoses, and treatments discussed in the book are for general information purposes only. They are not an exhaustive list of all possible situations for thyroid-related conditions or iodine imbalance scenarios.

Scientific knowledge about iodine's role in health is evolving, and new research may be available after the printing of this book. Always seek your doctor's guidance before taking any supplements or over-the-counter products.

Supplements are not well regulated by the Food and Drug Administration, and iodine content of different products can vary widely. Supplements may also interact with medications you may already be taking or cause side effects. Ask your doctor or pharmacist for more information about iodine supplements and proper dosages, if a supplement is recommended for you.

Introduction

Iodine has powerful effects on the body. It is a trace mineral that's necessary for your thyroid gland to make thyroid hormones. Thyroid hormones are vital for virtually every aspect of human development. If you're reading this book, you're likely curious about iodine's role in your own health.

There are plenty of websites, books, and videos discussing the effects of too little or too much iodine and how it impacts your health. Maybe you're wondering how this book is different. *The Iodine Balancing Handbook* takes a measured, evidence-based approach to explain why iodine is crucial for your health. The book will clearly explain facts about iodine's connection to normal thyroid function.

Iodine deficiency is still quite common in many parts of the world. Globally, studies indicate an estimated 50 million people show clinical signs of deficiency. Iodine is particularly important during pregnancy for fetal development. And iodine deficiency is recognized as the most common preventable cause of impaired brain development.[1] Changes in your iodine levels, including excess iodine, can disturb your thyroid function and cause thyroid-related disorders.

Iodine is a naturally occurring mineral that's found in soil and some bodies of water. Your diet, where you live, along with genetic, environmental, and even ethnocultural factors, can contribute to your iodine levels. Your body relies on external sources such as food, or dietary supplements, to meet its iodine needs. So, under-

---

1 B. G. Biban and C. Lichiardopol, "Iodine Deficiency, Still a Global Problem?" *Current Health Sciences Journal* 43, no. 2 (2017): 103–111, doi: 10.12865/CHSJ.43.02.01; Kahla Redman et al., "Iodine Deficiency and the Brain: Effects and Mechanisms," *Critical Reviews in Food Science and Nutrition* 56, no. 16 (2016): 2695–713, doi: 10.1080/10408398.2014.922042.

standing how your diet affects your thyroid function is crucial to maintaining balanced iodine levels.

If you're curious about the connection between iodine and your health, you've come to the right place for answers. The handbook outlines who is at risk for iodine imbalance, signs to look for, and what to do to manage an iodine imbalance. We'll explore why your body needs iodine and how shifts in iodine levels (up or down) affect your body.

Did you know that iodine needs are not constant? Throughout your life, your body's iodine requirements change to support development and growth. At certain times of your life, you need more iodine. For example, you need more iodine during pregnancy and while breastfeeding to support fetal and infant development.

In this book you'll find valuable information on common dietary sources of iodine, and how specific types of diets such as vegan diets may impact iodine levels long term. The book will also review age-based iodine guidelines and explore benefits of iodine balance for health and well-being.

There's a lot to understand about iodine, including its various forms and uses. There are differences between topical iodine, dietary supplements, prescription medications, and radioactive iodine (radioiodine), and in how each is used. In this book, we'll mainly focus on iodine's role for normal thyroid health.

The goal of this book is to increase your understanding about the significance of maintaining iodine sufficiency. We'll discuss when to talk with your doctor about checking your iodine levels and how to supplement iodine safely. If this has aroused your interest about this powerful micronutrient, dive in and learn more from *The Iodine Balancing Handbook*.

CHAPTER 1

Facts About Iodine

Key Points

- ✂ Iodine is an essential micronutrient required by the body to function normally.
- ✂ It is a nonmetallic halogen compound.
- ✂ Iodine is a mineral found naturally in soil, seawater, and rocks in trace amounts.
- ✂ The thyroid gland needs iodine to make thyroid hormones.

While you may not have given iodine much thought, there is a lot to appreciate about iodine's role in your everyday health. Your body needs this essential nutrient for your thyroid gland to produce thyroid hormones. You cannot produce iodine on your own—all the iodine your body needs must come from external sources such as the foods you eat. Yet, food sources of iodine are not constant or easy to measure, so it's difficult to gauge how much you're getting. This can lead to problems with your iodine levels in certain cases.

When you don't take in enough iodine, over time, you'll become iodine deficient. Conversely, if you take in too much iodine through certain foods, or by taking dietary supplements, this can also throw off the normal function of your thyroid gland. It's a delicate balance that's helpful to understand.

Changes in iodine levels can have a big impact on how well your thyroid gland works to produce thyroid hormones. If your iodine levels are off, you could develop thyroid disorders resulting from an over- or underactive thyroid. This can affect your energy, weight, metabolism, heart rate, blood pressure, and many other essential body functions.

Thyroid conditions such as goiter (enlarged thyroid gland) have been reported throughout history around the world. The discovery of iodine and its link to thyroid function and goiter was a major breakthrough.

In this chapter, we'll take a closer look at what iodine is and why we need it. We'll also discuss natural sources of iodine and explain how environmental changes around the world are contributing to unpredictable iodine levels in food sources.

What Is Iodine?

Iodine is a naturally occurring trace mineral that's found in some types of soil, rock formations, and saltwater bodies such as oceans and seas. It is a stable, nonmetallic halogen listed in the periodic table of elements as the symbol ①. Its atomic number is 53, and its atomic weight is 126.90.[2] It is the heaviest of the halogen elements. Some other common halogen elements include bromine, chlorine, and fluorine.

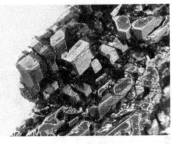

Elemental Iodine

Halogens have many useful properties that establish them as essential ingredients for products we use daily. Halogens react chemically with different elements, such as with hydrogen to make acids and with sodium to form salts.

The variety of halogens are used to make everything from household products (including paper), to cleaning products, to ingredients for types of industrial and pharmaceutical products, to food additives.

2 National Center for Biotechnology Information, "Iodine," *PubChem*, accessed September 7, 2022, https://pubchem.ncbi.nlm.nih.gov/compound/Iodine#section=Chemical-and-Physical-Properties.

For example, iodine reacts with sodium and potassium to form sodium iodide and potassium iodide. You're probably familiar with iodized salt. This is a common way iodine is added as a nutritional supplement to prevent iodine deficiency in the general population. We'll get into greater detail about how salt iodization was introduced to prevent iodine deficiency in chapter 2 on the history of iodine.

The solid form of iodine is grayish-black in color, and it has a strong, pungent odor. It is only slightly soluble in water. The liquid and vapor forms of iodine are deep purple in color. Iodine is dangerous in concentrated forms, and ingestion, inhalation, or skin contact can cause irritation, rash, burns, watery eyes, runny nose, headache, and other serious reactions.[3]

Iodine has many uses. It is well known for making dyes, in photography, and as a contrast agent for imaging such as computed tomography (CT) scans. It is also added to animal feed and used as a water purifier and a disinfectant. Topical iodine is an effective antiseptic and is useful for cleansing wounds. For example, a 1 percent iodine solution can kill 90 percent of bacteria on contact within 90 seconds.[4]

In this book, we'll focus mainly on the medical uses of iodine and the implications of iodine for your thyroid health.

Natural Sources of Iodine

Iodine is found in many natural sources such as soil, plants, water, and rocks. However, in nature, it is combined with other substances and is not free. These sources don't contain large amounts of the mineral, though. Higher amounts of natural iodine are mostly found in salt water such as oceans, but this is still not concentrated

3 National Center for Biotechnology Information, "Iodine."
4 National Center for Biotechnology Information, "Iodine."

⚖ The **Iodine Balancing** Handbook

enough for most commercial uses of iodine. Seaweed, sea sponges, and coral are good sources of natural iodine. Iodine for human consumption only makes up around 3 percent of the overall global iodine use.

As mentioned previously, iodine has many commercial uses. These require a much higher concentration of iodine than natural sources provide. For example, did you know that one of the most popular uses of iodine is for making contrast media for medical imaging products such as X-rays? In fact, 22 percent of iodine is used for this purpose alone.

Today most iodine for commercial use comes from underground oil brines in Japan and from a type of sedimentary rock called *caliche ores* in Chile.

Now, you're probably more curious about the best sources of iodine for human use. Where do we get the iodine to make thyroid hormones? Remember, our bodies cannot make iodine.

We rely mainly on food and supplement sources to get the iodine our body needs to avoid thyroid problems. Iodine is found in many types of foods we eat, but how much we get on a daily basis is not an exact science. Food sources of iodine can vary in quality depending on the soil where the food is grown, chemical processing, and food additives. Soil iodine content also varies based on its geographic region and other environmental factors. This is why, in 1993, the World Health Organization (WHO) and the United Nations Children's Fund (UNICEF) recommended that countries around the world add iodine to table salt as a simple way to lower risks of iodine deficiency and endemic goiter in human populations. But challenges and disparities remain with salt iodization globally. We'll discuss this later in the book.

Marine plants, such as kelp, and types of seafood, such as oysters and crustaceans, take in iodine from seawater or ocean water. These water-based food sources are some of the highest in iodine.

However, eating too much of these food types can cause iodine overload, increasing your risk for thyroid problems. Dairy products are another good dietary source of iodine. Yet, as with other food sources of iodine, the amounts of iodine found in various dairy products can vary a great deal. And those who avoid dairy run the increased risk of iodine deficiency if another good source is not substituted to maintain adequate levels.

In short, food grown in iodine-rich soil is the easiest way for us to get small amounts of daily iodine. The challenge is that environmental damage has reduced soil iodine levels in many areas. This particularly impacts mountainous regions and areas prone to frequent flooding. Crops that are grown in these types of soil don't contain much iodine. Over time, people living in these areas can develop iodine deficiency because they are not getting enough iodine through their diet. Plants typically are a poor source of iodine.

So, although you take in iodine from many different natural sources, the amount you're getting is difficult to gauge and may be inconsistent. Also, most natural food and drink sources of iodine don't contain enough to correct any major iodine deficiencies. On the other hand, eating too much of one type of iodine-rich food such as seaweed can lead to excessive iodine intake.

Around the world, over the past several centuries, environmental damage from flooding, soil erosion, and pesticide use have all stripped natural iodine levels.

While most people get the proper amount of iodine they need for normal thyroid function, some individuals are at increased risk of thyroid disorders. Without consistent dietary iodine, your thyroid will under- or overwork to make thyroid hormones. Both of these situations will cause multiple iodine-related health problems in the long term if they're not corrected.

Why Do We Need Iodine?

Your body needs iodine for normal growth, metabolism, and development for every stage of your life. Iodine is absorbed into your body through the stomach and small intestine and then transported to the thyroid gland. The thyroid gland is a tiny, butterfly-shaped organ that's located under the skin in the lower front area of your neck. The gland contains two lobes connected by a tissue band called an *isthmus*. These lobes have tiny sacs called *follicles* that store thyroid hormones. There are two different types of thyroid cells, called *follicular* and *parafollicular* cells.

The follicular thyroid cells are responsible for making the two main types of thyroid hormones: *thyroxine* (T4) and *triiodothyronine* (T3). T4 has four iodine atoms attached to it, and T3 has three iodine atoms attached to it. These hormones are part of your endocrine system. The endocrine system consists of glands in the body that make and release essential hormones to regulate your metabolism and cellular level activities.

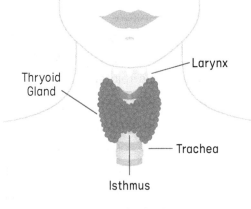

Thryoid Gland

Larynx

Trachea

Isthmus

Thyroid gland

The second type of thyroid cell tissue is called parafollicular cells or C-cells. These cells help make the hormone *calcitonin*. This hormone is responsible for regulating the amount of calcium and phosphate in your blood. Calcitonin helps with bone metabolism and other bodily processes.

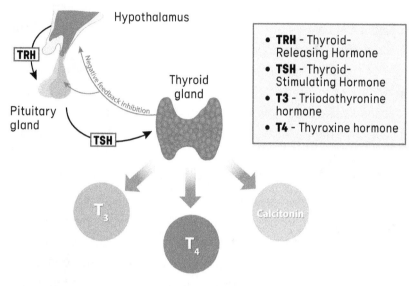

Thyroid hormones

Thyroid hormones are released into your bloodstream when they're needed for various cellular activities. They help regulate different body systems such as temperature, energy, and metabolism. For example, if your thyroid hormones don't work properly, you could feel tired, have trouble focusing, experience hair loss and dry skin, or have organ, bone, and muscle-related problems.

Your body's thyroid hormone needs change over time. How much is made and released depends on a complex signaling system in the brain. This is called a *continuous negative feedback loop* between the hypothalamus, the pituitary gland, and the thyroid gland.

When your body needs thyroid hormones, the hypothalamus sends a signal to release thyrotropin-releasing hormone, which then signals the pituitary gland to produce thyroid-stimulating hormone (TSH). This is a negative feedback loop. An increase in TSH tells the thyroid gland to make more thyroid hormones. Checking your blood TSH levels is one way your doctor can find out if your thyroid is working properly.

The thyroid gland uses the protein *thyroglobulin* to make T4 and T3 and to store iodine. Thyroglobulin is made in the thyroid gland follicles. Once TSH is released by your pituitary gland, your thyroid gland starts making T4, as well as T3 in smaller amounts. Even though your thyroid gland makes more T4, it is mostly inactive.

In order for the thyroid hormones to do their work at the cellular level, they must be activated. T4 is converted to the active form of thyroid hormone T3 with the help of certain enzymes (proteins) called *iodothyronine deiodinase*.[5] Currently, three deiodinase enzymes have been identified (DIO1, DIO2, DIO3) by scientists. They are found in different amounts in nearly every organ and tissue throughout the body.

Each has different functions. DIO1 is mainly responsible for converting T4 to active T3 in the thyroid gland and also to a lesser degree in the kidneys and liver. DIO2 is mainly responsible for producing T3 in cells all over the body including muscles, tissues, bones, and various organs. DIO3 is active during fetal development and protects tissues from too much thyroid hormone. And in adults, DIO3 is mostly present in skin and the central nervous system.

These enzymes are crucial for thyroid hormone signaling and regulation for normal growth and development. Although scientists aren't sure about the exact role of each type of deiodinase enzyme, they believe deiodinase enzymes are important in making sure thyroid hormone levels in the body, including at the cellular level, are stable. These enzymes allow tissues to decrease or increase thyroid hormone concentrations depending on cellular needs.[6]

5 Laura Sabatino et al., "Deiodinases and the Three Types of Thyroid Hormone Deiodination Reactions," *Endocrinology and Metabolism* 36, no. 5 (2021): 952–64, doi: 10.3803/EnM.2021.1198.0.1038/s41574-019-0218-2.

6 Sabatino et al., "Deiodinases and the Three Types of Thyroid Hormone Deiodination Reactions."

In order to make thyroid hormones, the gland needs sufficient levels of circulating iodide, which you get from your diet as either iodide, iodate, or organically bound iodine taken as supplements.

The amount of iodine you need changes and depends on your age. Pregnant women and breastfeeding mothers need the highest amounts of iodine to support not only their own health but also the health of their unborn babies.

How much iodine a pregnant woman takes in is critical for the health of her growing baby; iodine is essential for normal fetal development. In parts of the world where iodine is low in soil and water sources, pregnant women can develop serious iodine deficiency, which can affect brain development and cause other iodine-related disorders in their babies. This has lifelong consequences.

Iodine Versus Iodide

You'll read about iodine and iodide throughout this book, and you may wonder about the difference between these terms. While they're not interchangeable, they are closely related.

Iodine is an element available in trace amounts in nature. As mentioned, it has an atomic number of 53, and it is the heaviest of the halogen compounds. It has a neutral electron charge and is not easily soluble in water. Iodine on its own is very corrosive and can cause burns, irritation, and damage to skin and tissues with direct contact. It is typically bonded with another chemical entity for use in humans.

Iodide is a different chemical entity of iodine. It is a negatively charged ion molecule of iodine. It is formed when iodine combines with a positively charged element such as potassium or sodium to form a salt such as potassium iodide or sodium iodide.

Salt forms of iodine are more stable, and most types of iodine supplements contain potassium iodide. Iodized salt was introduced as a simple and an inexpensive way to lower rates of goiter and severe iodine deficiency around the world. Once iodide is ingested, the body has to break it down into iodine for it to be used.

Lugol's solution was developed in the early 1800s, combining iodine, potassium iodide, and distilled water. It was used for many different medical treatments, including as an antiseptic and to treat iodine deficiency. It is still available in generic versions today in various strengths.

Potassium iodide supplements come in different strengths and formulations. These are used to treat iodine deficiency, used as a diagnostic agent to detect cancerous cells, and also used to block radioactive iodine from being absorbed by the thyroid gland.

In a nuclear disaster, such as from a nuclear power plant, radio-active iodine in the environment may be absorbed into the body, causing radiation poisoning. High levels of radioactive iodine in the body can increase the risk for thyroid cancer, especially in infants, children, and adolescents. When potassium iodide is taken, ideally before exposure to radioactive iodine, the thyroid gland absorbs the potassium iodide and it blocks radioactive iodine from being taken up by the gland. Consequently, potassium iodide has a protecting effect.

Potassium iodide only offers protection against radioactive iodine, not other forms of radiation exposure. Not everyone can take this form of iodide, and its use is limited to specific situations. When used for radioactive iodine exposure, it is typically only used in people 40 years and younger. To be effective in protecting the thyroid gland, it has to be given 24 hours before an exposure or within four hours of radioactive iodine exposure. It doesn't provide complete protection. It is not recommended for use without medical consultation.

CHAPTER 2

The History of Iodine and the Thyroid Gland

Key Points

- ✗ Iodine was discovered in 1811.
- ✗ Endemic goiter refers to swelling of the thyroid gland from iodine deficiency in a population.
- ✗ The function of the thyroid gland wasn't understood until the early nineteenth century.
- ✗ Swiss physician Jean-François Coindet first used iodine in the 1820s to treat goiter.
- ✗ Universal salt iodization began in the 1920s in the United States.

The French chemist Bernard Courtois accidentally discovered iodine in 1811 in the process of making gunpowder during the Napoleonic Wars. Courtois was originally using wood ash to make saltpeter (potassium nitrate), a key ingredient used in gunpowder. Later, due to the low supply of wood in the area, he switched to using seaweed ash, which was more abundantly available to him.

One day he noticed a violet-colored vapor forming when he used too much sulfuric acid to wash the copper vessels he was using. The vapor then condensed into crystals. Courtois believed he had discovered a new compound, but because of the war, he didn't have the resources to study it.

Courtois decided to give samples of the substance to chemists he knew to help identify the compound. While there is historical debate about who actually first identified the element iodine, there is agreement that Courtois first discovered it.

Several chemists, including Charles-Bernard Désormes, Nicolas Clément, Joseph Louis Gay-Lussac, and André M. Ampère, studied the crystals and reported they had found a new compound or element. Historical accounts say Gay-Lussac named the new element "iode" from the Greek name for violet "*ioeides*." Around the same time, a British chemist, Sir Humphry Davy, also published a report based on his experiments that the new element was similar to chlorine and fluorine. Historical accounts suggest he named it "iodine" to keep the name consistent with the other halogen elements chlorine and fluorine.[7]

As we touched upon earlier, iodine is only slightly water soluble. That means it doesn't easily dissolve unless it's mixed with another agent or a mineral such as potassium or chlorine. In 1829, French physician Jean Guillaume Auguste Lugol (1788–1851) discovered bonding iodine with potassium allowed it to dissolve in water. He was studying treatments for tuberculosis and thought iodine solution would be an effective one.

He developed "Lugol's solution," consisting of a 1:2 ratio made up of one part elemental iodine and two parts potassium iodide mixed with distilled water. Although Lugol's solution was not effective for tuberculosis, it was an effective treatment for iodine-related thyroid gland problems. Lugol's solution is still available in generic versions today. It is used in various strengths as preparation before thyroid surgery, and to treat various types of thyroid conditions such as an overactive thyroid gland. It works by reducing the size of the thyroid gland and how much thyroid hormone it produces.

7 Angela M. Leung, Lewis E. Braverman, and Elizabeth N. Pearce, "History of U.S. Iodine Fortification and Supplementation," *Nutrients* 4, no. 11 (2012): 1740–46, doi: 10.3390/nu4111740.

But the discovery of iodine wasn't the beginning of the story. Modern medical understanding of thyroid disorders, including endemic goiter related to iodine deficiency, is based on the evolution of medical science going back thousands of years. Centuries before iodine's connection to thyroid health was established, philosophers, artists, physicians, and anatomists proposed various theories about the thyroid gland and its function in a person's health.

Sadly, during many ancient eras, because goiter was not well understood, the physical appearance from swelling had negative connotations. In paintings, frescoes, sculptures, and books that we can still view, people with goiter were depicted in a negative light as executioners, mentally unstable, or "evil."

However, examining these records also provides us with a fascinating look into how each era classified thyroid disorders and contributed toward shifts in beliefs and medical practice for future generations. Each subsequent generation built on the progress of the past to improve medical care.

Endemic Iodine Deficiency

Goiter, which is an enlarged thyroid gland, was endemic in many regions of the world before iodine treatment was established. Goiter may be caused by different problems with thyroid function including inflammatory conditions of the thyroid gland. However, goiter caused by iodine deficiency in a region, is referred to as endemic goiter.[8] Although iodine's role in treating goiter was unknown for hundreds of years, iodine-rich foods still played a role in various treatments throughout history.

Written descriptions and illustrations of goiter and other thyroid-related conditions are as varied as the geographic regions of the

---

8 Ahmet S. Can and Anis Rehman, "Goiter," in *StatPearls* (Treasure Island, FL: StatPearls Publishing, 2022).

world from which they were reported. Many medical treatises and explanations were influenced by religious and philosophical beliefs of the time. Hypotheses over the ages were sometimes cohesive, but more often they were conflicting, adding to confusion in detection and treatment of thyroid conditions for hundreds of years. But regardless of the assumptions about its origins, global historical records show that goiter was present from the earliest days of human history.

Around the world, goiter was more common in areas where the soil content of iodine was especially low. But the link between soil mineral content (iodine) and endemic thyroid disorder wasn't made until the mid-1800s. In America, goiter was primarily endemic in the Midwest, the Appalachian region, the Great Lakes, and the Inter-mountain Region.

Geographically, soil levels of iodine were also low in parts of China, India, places in Central Africa and Central Asia, and mountainous regions including Switzerland, the Andes, and the Himalayas.

A few of these geographic regions of the world such as Central Africa continue to have iodine deficiency among the population. They are some of the areas where thyroid-related disorders among infants, young children, and pregnant and breastfeeding women are the most prevalent today.

Medical Discovery of the Thyroid Gland

The earliest written records from around 3600 BC, Chinese documents, describe people with goiter.[9] Indian Ayurvedic medicine dating back to 1400 BC also offers detailed descriptions of *"galaganda,"* or goiter. Ayurvedic texts also made references

---

9 Leung et al., "History of U.S. Iodine Fortification."

to different thyroid conditions in distinct categories: *kaphaja* (hypothyroidism), *vataja* (hyperthyroidism), and *medaja* (thyroidal cyst). Historical records from Egypt around 1500 BC also discuss people with goiter.

The earliest surviving graphical sketches of thyroid disorders are thought to be from an illustration in a book titled *Reuner Musterbuch*, from around 1215 AD. The text was from a Cistercian abbey in the Alps. Prior to the start of salt iodization programs in the 1920s, Switzerland had a large number of people affected by goiter.

The images linked the thyroid conditions goiter and "cretinism"—an ancient term used to describe people with impaired physical and mental development from hypothyroidism. The conditions were not well understood at the time.[10] Severe iodine deficiency in pregnant women caused goiter and cretinism, or developmental disabilities, in infants, but the connection was not established for many hundreds of years.

Around the fifteenth and sixteenth centuries, the beginning of the Western Renaissance period, several prominent anatomists, artists, and physicians identified the thyroid gland. However, its function still remained a mystery until the early nineteenth century.

In earlier times, many believed the gland served a structural role. Historians believe Leonardo da Vinci first drew an anatomical image of the thyroid gland around 1511, but he thought its purpose was to hold the trachea in place and fill the gap between the neck muscles.[11]

Andreas Vesalius (1514–1564) was a Belgian doctor and anatomist who published the first illustrated book on human anatomy, called

---

10 Asfandyar Khan Niazi et al., "Thyroidology Over the Ages," *Indian Journal of Endocrinology and Metabolism* 15, no. 2 (2011): S121–S126, doi: 10.4103/2230-8210 .83347.

11 D. Lydiatt and G. Bucher, "Historical Vignettes of the Thyroid Gland," *Clinical Anatomy* 24, no. 1 (2010): 1-9.

De Humani Corporis Fabrica Libri Septem or *Fabrica*. In the book he described and illustrated the thyroid gland.

Then, in the seventeenth century, Thomas Wharton (1614–1673), an English physician and anatomist, authored *Adenographia*. It became the most well-known and respected book classifying the various glands of the body, including naming the thyroid gland "*Glandulae thyreoidea*." The book was so popular it was reprinted six times and was used for over two hundred years. It also set off considerable debate and speculation about the function of the thyroid gland well into the twentieth century.[12]

There were other well-known physicians from the eighteenth and nineteenth centuries who had observed goiter and *exophthalmos* (bulging eyes) and reported their findings. They included the English physician Caleb Parry (1755–1822), Irish physician Robert Graves (1796–1853), and German physician Carl von Basedow Merseburg (1799–1854). They independently described prominent swelling of the thyroid gland with palpitations and bulging eyes (symptoms known as the "Merseburg Triad"). The term *Graves' disease* is named after Robert Graves, based on his work on the thyroid gland—the phrase appeared in medical literature from 1862.[13]

Theories on Causes of Goiter

The origin of the word "goiter" or "goitre" may have come from the old French word *goitron*, meaning throat, or the Latin word for *guttur*, which also refers to throat. Although goiter was endemic in many parts of the world, its cause was misunderstood for hundreds of years. Over time, theories ranged from evil spirits to natural phenomena being responsible.

---

12 K. Laios et al., "From Thyroid Cartilage to Thyroid Gland," *Folia Morphologica* 78, no. 1 (2019): 171–73, doi: 10.5603/FM.a2018.0059.

13 V. C. Medvei, *A History of Endocrinology* (Lancaster, England: MTP Press, 1982), 289-96.

While it's impossible to dig into every notion or philosophy proposed over thousands of years, let's take a look at a few notable contributions to give you an idea of the vast scope of scientific discovery through generations of research, observation, and practice. After all, the foundation of modern medicine and scientific achievements are all grounded in history.

Hippocrates (460–370 BC), who is often referred to as the "Father of Medicine" in the Western world, wrote extensively about various ailments and infectious diseases. He advocated that natural phenomena were responsible for diseases, rather than magical or supernatural forces. At the time, this was not the majority belief. However, Hippocrates was well respected during his lifetime, and his medical discourses were embraced for centuries.

In his book from 400 BC titled *On Airs, Waters, and Places*, he described goiter as being caused by "drinking snow water." He thought the function of the thyroid gland was to lubricate respiratory passages. Hippocrates also believed natural sources—soil, water, and air—influenced disease. He thought health was achieved through the balance between body fluids and external forces (nature), and if this balance was disordered, it led to illness.[14]

Although rudimentary in its premise, the concept of natural sources influencing disease still holds true today. For example, we only need to consider how environmental toxins in soil, air, and water negatively affect our health globally to appreciate Hippocrates's philosophy. Separately, his philosophies and ethical standards regarding the practice of medicine are still valid and adhered to by physicians today.

Another well-respected Greek physician, surgeon, and philosopher, Galen (129–216 AD), also made major contributions to medical practice. However, he disagreed with previous theories proposed

---

14 Hippocrates, translated by Francis Adams, *On Airs, Waters, and Places* (London: Wyman & Sons, 1881).

⚖️ The **Iodine Balancing** Handbook

by other physicians about the role of the thyroid. Galen believed it served as a link and a shield between the brain and the heart.

His scientific impact includes helping to increase understanding of the circulatory system and the glands of the body. Galen thought the purpose of the thyroid gland was to absorb nerve impulses from the circulatory system. His observations and theories on anatomy, and the causes and treatments for various illnesses, were generally accepted and recognized until the sixteenth century.

Other global historical records point to water as a potential cause for goiter. The ancient Chinese attributed goiter to living in mountainous regions and poor-quality water. The Swiss physician Philippus Theophrastus Aureolus Bombastus von Hohenheim, who went by the name Paracelsus, described goiter and cretinism caused by minerals in water, particularly lead.

Over time, a few common rationales emerged regarding possible causes of goiter. They included properties of water; climatic causes such as temperature, lack of sun, and humidity; and social and medical causes such as poverty, poor nutrition, insanity, and poor living conditions. There were also differences that emerged between American scientists and European scientists.

One American physician and botanist, Benjamin Smith Barton (1766–1815), wrote a book in the year 1800 addressed to a colleague at the University of Göttingen in Germany titled *A Memoir Concerning the Disease of Goitre as It Prevails in Different Parts of North America.*[15]

Barton called out distinct geographic differences between European mountainous and American nonmountainous regional cases of goiter, their causes, and cures based on his travels and observations. He wrote, "As the disease of goitre is extremely common in some parts of Germany, and in other parts of Europe,

---

15 Sarah E. Naramore, "Making Endemic Goiter an American Disease, 1800–1820," *Journal of the History of Medicine and Allied Science* 76, no. 3 (2021): 239–63, doi: 10 .1093/jhmas/jrab018.

the philosophical physicians of those countries will not deem it an incurious point to examine with attention, what affinity there is between the soil, the climates and exposure to the European districts in which this disease prevails, and the soil, the climates and exposure of those countries in [North] America in which it also prevails."[16]

Barton expressed his regret that he didn't have much new information to contribute but hoped the book would generate interest for others to learn more. He wrote, "I know that the path to temporary glory leads through the fairy-land of theory: but the road to present and to future usefulness lies through the field of facts and observation."[17] But Barton, like others before him, hypothesized that "goitre is a *miasm* of the same species as that which produces intermittent and remittent fevers, dysentery and familiar complaints."[18] This was a popular theory for hundreds of years.

Barton's memoir provides a captivating glimpse into his thoughts behind health and illness related to the thyroid gland from over two hundred years ago.[19]

The popular hypothesis that goiter may be caused by an infection persisted for many years in different parts of the world. For example, Theodor Billroth (1829–1894), a well-respected and skilled Austrian surgeon, believed goiter was caused by "miasmatic tumors" and "local expressions of general infection." This was similar to Barton's theory on the cause for goiter. The infection theory continued into the nineteenth century.

In 1878, physician William Ord, who was affiliated with St. Thomas Hospital in London, first used the term "myxoedema" to describe

---

16 Benjamin Smith Barton, *A Memoir Concerning the Disease of Goitre as It Prevails in Different Parts of North America* (Philadelphia, PA: Way & Groff, 1800).

17 Benjamin Smith Barton, A Memoir Concerning the Disease of Goitre.

18 Benjamin Smith Barton, A Memoir Concerning the Disease of Goitre.

19 You can read more here: https://archive.org/details/b30794808/page/2/mode/2up?ref=ol&view=theater.

⚖ **The Iodine Balancing** Handbook

hypothyroidism. He wrote a paper titled "On Myxoedema, a Term Proposed to Be Applied to an Essential Condition in the 'Cretinoid' Affection Occasionally Observed in Middle-Aged Women," in which he described the thyroid condition as a "mucous oedema" of the skin.[20]

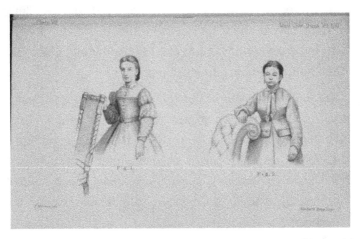

This photo is the first lithographic image of a young woman with thyroid deficiency. It shows the change over seven years, from when she was 21 years old (left image). The photos appeared in Ord's paper from 1878.[21]

In 1909, Swiss physician Emil Theodor Kocher (1841–1917) received the Nobel Prize in physiology and medicine for his many contributions toward understanding thyroid function, disorder, and surgery along with his work on other endocrine disorders. Kocher believed iodine was important for thyroid function, but he was not able to prove it scientifically during his lifetime.

20 Stefan Slater, "The Discovery of Thyroid Replacement Therapy," *JLL Bulletin: Commentaries on the History of Treatment Evaluation*, jameslindlibrary.org/articles /the-discovery-of-thyroid-replacement-therapy.

21 William M. Ord, "On Myxoedema, a Term Proposed to Be Applied to an Essential Condition in the 'Cretinoid' Affection Occasionally Observed in Middle-Aged Women," *Medio-Chiurological Transactions*, no. 61 (1878): 57–78.5, doi: 10.1177/09595287780610 0107.

It was Eugen Baumann (1846–1896), a German chemist and professor of medicine, who was the first to report, in 1895, that iodine was a natural component of thyroid tissue.

In America, there were exciting developments in medicine that occurred in the early twentieth century. A popular paper authored by two renowned physicians, Charles H. Mayo and Henry W. Plummer, titled "The Thyroid Gland" discussed the anatomy, physiology, function, and diseases of the thyroid. The paper delves into various historical theories on the causes of goiter.

Mayo and Plummer wrote about the dominant theories including "inorganic and organic chemicals found in the water," "a toxic infective theory," "the lack of iodin in the food," and "general hygiene." They also discussed common infectious diseases of childhood such as measles, mumps, whooping cough, and other illnesses causing chronic (long-standing) inflammation leading to thyroid imbalance.

They say that "chronic debilitating diseases exert a harmful influence on the thyroid partly due to their impairment of nutrition and partly due to the toxic action of the products of their causal agents which result in a depreciation of the thyroid's reserve store of energy." They go on to say that "it is thought probable that the slight fullness of the neck, to which they occasionally give rise, is due normally, to the increased flow of blood to the gland occasioned by its increased physiologic action." The paper provides an account of historical discoveries regarding iodine's role in thyroid function, along with observations and speculation from Mayo and Plummer about causes of goiter based on their knowledge at the time.[22]

Mayo and Plummer wrote that endemic goiter was caused by iodine deficiency which affected normal thyroid function. They went on

---

22 Charles H. Mayo and Henry W. Plummer, "The Thyroid Gland," Wellcome Collection, https://wellcomecollection.org/works/r3x9xckc/items?canvas=2.

to say that water and food iodine levels were the main causes of endemic goiter in populations.

Over centuries, many different theories for goiter were touted by various philosophers and physicians, but it wasn't until the 1940s that scientific evidence identified iodine deficiency as the root cause of endemic goiter.

Ancient Treatments for Goiter

Prior to the discovery of iodine's role in thyroid function, different cures and treatments were recommended for goiter and thyroid conditions, including surgery. Some food-based solutions were remarkably effective due to their high iodine content.

The Ayurvedic physician Acharya Charaka, born in 300 BC, described hypothyroidism and how to prevent the condition. He felt a person's lifestyle and environment influenced their health and wellness. Ayurveda is based on the belief that the universe is composed of five elements (air, fire, water, earth, and space), and health is the balance between mind, body, and spirit.

Charaka suggested consuming adequate amounts of barley, rice, milk, cucumber, sugarcane juice, and green grams (mung beans) to counteract goiter. Dairy foods have adequate iodine content, and with daily consumption, would have improved mild or moderate deficiency iodine deficiency. We'll discuss iodine content of different types of food in chapter 7.

Galen recommended using burnt sea sponge to treat goiters in 150 AD. Various Chinese treatments dating back from around 300 AD described using seaweed, sargassum, and burnt sea sponges. In 650 AD, the Chinese physician Sun Simiao wrote about using chopped animal thyroid gland, ground mollusk shells, seaweed, and burnt sea sponges to treat goiter. Again, these are some of the highest sources of iodine.

From around 400 AD until the 1400s, several prominent physicians wrote encyclopedic texts on various diseases and their treatments. Among them were various surgical procedures to treat goiter.

Unfortunately, in ancient times, goiter surgery, when attempted, caused serious complications and had high death rates. This was because of rudimentary instruments; poor understanding of the circulatory system, which led to postsurgery hemorrhaging; and infections, among other difficulties.

A renowned Byzantine physician, Aëtius of Amida (527–564 AD), may have been the first to document goiter and exophthalmos (thyroid eye disease) in a patient. He worked in Constantinople in the court of Emperor Justinian I. Aëtius is credited with writing a set of medical practice books: Sixteen Books on Medicine.[23] Many of them contain information already established by earlier famous Greek physicians such as Galen. But Aëtius also provided detailed original work based on his medical experience of different conditions of the skin, eyes, ears, nose, and throat. In the books, he discussed various treatments and surgical procedures, which were used by physicians in later time periods. Among his recorded surgical procedures, he described surgery to relieve goiter, which he believed was a hernia affecting the larynx. He also mistakenly believed exophthalmos was a form of aneurysm (which is an abnormal swelling of the wall of a blood vessel).

In the seventh century, another famous Greek physician and surgeon, Paul of Aegina (625–690 AD), wrote a set of books Epitomoe Medicae Libri Septem (Medical Compendium in Seven Books). His work was based on medical practices of previous prominent Greek physicians including Galen, Oribasius, and Aëtius of Amida.[24]

---

23 D. Lazaris, F. Laskaratos, and G. Lascaratos, "Surgical Diseases of the Womb According to Aëtius of Amida (6th Century A.D.)," *World Journal of Surgery*, 33(6) (2009): 1310–17.

24 K. Jang, J. V. Rosenfeld, and A. Di leva, "Paulus of Aegina and the Historical Origins of Spine Surgery," *World Neurosurgery*, 133 (2020): 291–301.

The sixth book in the series he wrote is dedicated to surgical practices. In it, he describes surgical procedures including tracheotomy, tonsillectomy, and thyroidectomy. However, he mistakenly believed goiter was caused by *"bronchocele,"* a tumor of the neck.[25] Removal of the thyroid posed many dangers since the cause of goiter and the function of the thyroid gland was not understood. Surgery was a last option when breathing became difficult due to the size of the goiter.

Abu Al Qasim Khalaf Ibn Abbas Al Zahrawi, known as Albucasis (1013–1106), is credited with performing the first thyroidectomy (removal of thyroid).[26] He described goiter as "elephantiasis of the throat."

In 1170 AD, Roger of Palermo prescribed ashes of sponges and seaweed as a moderate way to treat goiter. However, he did recommend using surgery if it became necessary.

Until the fifteenth century, physicians around the globe experimented with and proposed many different treatments to treat goiter, including using animal thyroid, seaweed, and topical ointments. Some treatments had success, while others, such as surgery, often led to patients dying. In some cases, various nutritional treatments made their condition worse, because there was a lack of understanding about the fundamental role of the thyroid gland and how iodine balance worked.

I hope the glimpse back in time, reviewing the history of medical discovery made over thousands of years, helps explain why medicine is considered both an art and a science. Even today, the evolution of medical innovation takes years and often involves multiple detours. But despite all the breakthroughs, until the nineteenth century, experts were still in the dark about the thyroid–iodine connection.

25 Dimitrios Papapostolou et al., "Paul of Aegina (ca 625–690 AD): Operating on All, from Lymph Nodes in the Head and Neck to Visceral Organs in the Abdomen," *Cureus* 12, no. 3 (2020): e7287, doi: 10.7759/cureus.7287.

26 Samir S. Amr and Abdelghani Tbakhi, "Abu Al Qasim Al Zahrawi (Albucasis): Pioneer of Modern Surgery," *Annals of Saudi Medicine* 27, no. 3 (2007): 220–221, doi: 10.5144/0256-4947.2007.220.

Establishing the Iodine Connection

In the 1800s and early 1900s, there was much progress toward understanding thyroid function and the role of iodine. A Swiss physician, Jean-François Coindet (1774–1834), had a theory that iodine might improve goiter symptoms based on published information that iodine was a component of sea sponges and seaweed.

At the time, the cause of goiter was still unclear, but Coindet suspected there was a connection to iodine. He wrote a set of three memoirs in 1820 detailing his findings. The papers were titled "Observations on the Remarkable Effects of Iodine in Bronchocele and Schrophula."

In ancient times "scrofula" referred to tuberculosis infection occurring outside the lungs. Coindet wrote, "The bronchocele or goitre, is, for the most part, an indolent tumour, formed by the development of the thyroid gland occupying its centre, either of its lobes, or even its entire substance." He went on: "It is an organ whose use is unknown . . . . By the use of iodine, I have known a patient, at first relieved, and shortly after cured, when nearly suffocated."[27]

Coindet admitted that he didn't know the cause of goiter, yet he rejected previous historical "erroneous hypotheses, or to conjectures." Instead, he offered his own theories in his memoir. He said that "two different causes have, in my opinion, produced the goitre at Geneva; the first which is occasioned by the use of hard water, or the pump water of the lower streets in the city, brings on the goitre very speedily . . . this form of the disease, rarely of any moment, passes readily away on changing the drink."

---

27 J. F. Coindet, *Observations on the Remarkable Effects of Iodine in Bronchocele and Schrophula* (London: Paternoster-Row, 1821).

He continued: "The second is connected with causes that may be considered as mechanical and local—others as physiological; the former are produced by the effect of a laborious parturition, vomiting, coughing, crying, anger, or by the custom of the women in this place bearing heavy burthens upon their heads; they affect, more especially, the lower class of society."

His speculations on the causes of goiter continued: "In many cases it is developed on the approach of the critical age; chagrin, nervous attacks, moral affections, also contribute to its formation. These different circumstances explain, why in the adult age the goitre is much more frequent among women than men."

Coindet explained that iodine content in sea sponges is too small to determine a quantity to use. He created different strengths of iodine solutions mixed with water, wine, or syrup to treat goiter. At first, he started using 6 to 10 drops of iodine mixed with water taken three times a day, gradually increasing the dose up to 20 drops three times a day, or decreasing the dose as needed.

Coindet reported giving iodine solution to his patients with goiter, and he found it helped to reduce the size of the goiter. His work was translated into English by his friend and physician J. R. Johnson, and the treatment grew in popularity. However, the success of his treatment was mixed.

Coindet strongly believed in iodine's effectiveness and safety for the treatment of goiter, but he started hearing of dangerous side effects with its use. When he heard this, he wrote in his memoir, "As among 150 patients to whom I have administered iodine, or its different preparations, not one who has regularly and strictly followed my advice, has been exposed (at least to any great degree) to the disastrous effects attributed to it."

He told colleagues, "I had no doubt, that iodine, if injudiciously administered, would produce some distressing symptoms." Coindet advocated for iodine solution not to be available for sale to the public in pharmacies. Instead, he recommended only a physician or surgeon should prescribe it to patients. But while Coindet urged caution in using iodine solution for goiter, it was available over the counter in many towns, so people started using large doses. This led to serious side effects such as heart palpitations, weight loss, tremors, and other negative health effects associated with too much iodine and thyroid problems.

These serious reactions were due to excess iodine causing hyperthyroidism, an unrecognized medical condition at the time. Unfortunately, the widespread reports of bad reactions led to iodine being viewed as poisonous. In his third memoir, Coindet proposed using iodine in an ointment form to reduce side effects associated with drinking iodine solution.

However, this form of iodine was not effective and was soon abandoned. Coindet also used iodine for many other types of conditions including "dropsy," syphilis, "enlarged glands of the breast," "certain affections of the uterus," and more. But he lost his credibility, and physicians were skeptical of iodine's benefits. They felt it was harmful and stopped using it. This was a major setback in the treatment of iodine deficiency.

Chemist Jean-Baptiste Boussingault (1801–1887) believed a bad substance in the water caused goiter and cretinism. He had broad training and experience in chemistry, climatology, geology, medicine, and several other areas. He gained practical knowledge through his work in many diverse disciplines, such as mining, in his travels. He had seen goiter in the Alsace region where he worked in his early years, and during his travels in Venezuela and Colombia in South America. He noticed that people in certain areas of South America, such as Cartago in the Cauca Valley, didn't have goiter while in other areas, such as Mariquita and Santa Fe de Bogotá, it was endemic among women and even in dogs.

In a paper published in 1833, he wrote that the people of Cartago in Antioquia, Colombia, didn't have goiter because they consumed a "certain amount of iodine" daily from the salt available in that region. He went on to say that goiter would disappear if the government allowed everyone to have access to iodized salt.

Boussingault advocated using iodized salt in foods, which "is always followed by happy results" and cautioned against using iodine alone because it could have dangerous consequences. However, he never linked the lack of iodine to goiter or cretinism; instead he thought goiter was caused by drinking water that was composed of insufficient air.

In 1852, a French chemist, Gaspard Adolphe Chatin (1813–1901), published his theory that iodine found in certain freshwater plants and burnt sea sponges could be used to treat iodine deficiency, which caused goiter. He also suggested using iodine to treat scrofula from tuberculosis and other conditions caused by inflammation of tissues.

In 1883, Sir Felix Semon, a physician at St. Thomas Hospital in London, asserted that *cachexia strumipriva*, cretinism, and myxedema were all caused by disorder or absence of the thyroid.[28]

In 1891, George Redmayne Murray decided to experiment with subcutaneous (under the skin) injections of thyroid extract from sheep to treat hypothyroidism. He based this treatment on previous experiments with sheep thyroid transplants by Antonio Maria Bettencourt Rodrigues and José António Serrano of Lisbon. He wrote that "it seems reasonable to suppose that the same amount of improvement might be obtained by simply injecting the juice or an extract of the thyroid gland of a sheep beneath the skin of the patient."[29]

---

28 Stefan Slater, "The Discovery of Thyroid Replacement Therapy; Part 3: A Complete Transformation," *Journal of the Royal Society of Medicine* 104, no. 3 (2011): 100–106, doi: 10.1258/jrsm.2010.10k052.

29 Slater, "The Discovery of Thyroid Replacement Therapy."

He provided detailed descriptions of the process of extracting the sheep thyroid and injecting the thyroid juice extract under the "loose skin of the back, between the shoulder blades" of the patient. His experiments had mixed success with some positive and some negative results. However, his scientific experiments were published in the prestigious *British Medical Journal* and gained some popularity for his studies. But because two of his patients died after the injections, medical scientists urged caution with the treatment.

In 1895, Eugen Baumann discovered iodine in thyroid tissue of both animals and humans. This was the early point of discovery connecting iodine to thyroid function, which ultimately linked low iodine levels with poor thyroid function. In 1914, Edward C. Kendall isolated the pure form of thyroxine crystals from the thyroid gland. This was a scientific breakthrough in proving the iodine–thyroid connectivity research.

Iodization of common salt to counter iodine deficiency began in the 1920s. Initially, it started in the United States and Switzerland where rates of endemic goiter were as high as 70 percent in some areas, before it was adopted by other parts around Europe. In fact, goiter was so common in certain parts of the US, in 1918 before the US entered World War I, the Michigan draft board rejected more than 30 percent of recruits due to goiter and other serious thyroid conditions.

In 1917, physician David Marine and his team of researchers from Ohio started an iodine supplementation study. They gave one group of adolescent girls 9 milligrams (mg) per day of iodine to study how it affected goiter. They reported that those who received iodine had a reduction in goiter size compared with those who did not receive iodine.

In 1922, David Cowie, a physician from Michigan, speaking at a thyroid symposium for the Michigan State Medical Society, proposed that the United States should start a salt iodization program to address simple goiter. Together, Cowie and the society formed the Iodized Salt Committee, which ultimately led to routine salt iodization in the United States.

Unfortunately, the road to universal salt iodization was a rocky one. Routine iodine supplementation was not easily accepted due to worries over its safety and unclear public health messaging about the need for iodine.

It took several years of lobbying salt companies, and many meetings around the state with prominent physicians, to convince them of the health benefits of iodized salt to prevent thyroid problems. Finally, in May of 1924, salt companies agreed.

Several months later, the Morton Salt company based in Chicago started adding iodine to its salt and distributing it nationwide.[30]

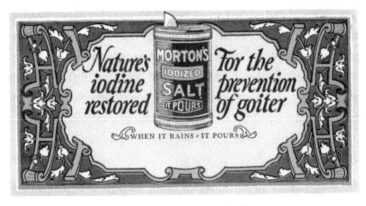

Morton Salt company 1925 advertisement. Photo credit: University of Michigan Center for the History of Medicine.

The dose of iodized salt commercially available in 1924 in Michigan was 100 milligrams (mg) per kilogram (kg) of salt. This resulted in an average daily iodine intake of 500 micrograms (µg). The amount of iodine in common table salt has evolved over the past 100 years.

30 Howard Markel, "A Grain of Salt," *The Milbank Quarterly* 92, no. 3 (2014): 407–12, doi: 10.1111/1468-0009.12064.

A few years after salt iodization began, in 1926, physician C. L. Hartsock and colleagues reported an increase in hyperthyroidism (overactive thyroid gland). In a paper titled "Iodized Salt in the Prevention of Goiter: Is It a Safe Measure for General Use?" they concluded it was caused by consuming iodized salt.[31]

Hartsock wrote that "the accumulated evidence seems to point conclusively to the continued ingestion of small amounts of iodine in the insidious form of iodized salt as the primary exciting factor. For this reason, we feel that it is important to call the attention of physicians, and through them of the public, to the misunderstanding that has gradually arisen regarding the use of iodine in endemic goiter, particularly in the form of iodized salt. Without any precaution being given for its use, this salt is being vigorously promoted by the combined propaganda of health officials and of salt companies."[32]

Once again, public health officials, physicians, and the public became concerned about routine iodine use, creating skepticism about its benefits in preventing iodine deficiency and goiter. Iodine supplementation in salt was not widely accepted around the world for many decades after it was proposed because of the cost, and in some areas, an increase in cases of hyperthyroidism, also known as Jod-Basedow syndrome, caused by excess iodine intake due to unclear standards on appropriate dosages of iodine for routine daily use.

By the way, the need for iodine supplementation and appropriate daily intake is still being debated today!

By 1935, rates of goiter had dropped appreciably by 74 to 90 percent in Michigan, especially among children who used iodized salt for at least six months. It also started dropping in other parts of the country once people started buying iodized salt.

---

31 C. L. Hartsock, "Iodized Salt in the Prevention of Goiter: Is It a Safe Measure for General Use?" *Journal of the American Medical Association* 86, no. 18 (1926): 1334–38, doi: 10.1001/Jama.1926.02670440008005.

32 Hartsock, "Iodized Salt."

Efforts to mandate salt iodization nationwide through legislation proposed by the US Endemic Goiter Committee in 1948 failed. However, since the 1950s, it is estimated that around 70–76 percent of American households use iodized salt exclusively.

Today, a typical one-pound container of iodized salt contains 68 mcg (micrograms) of iodine in one-quarter teaspoon of salt, which provides about 45 percent of the daily value of iodine.

Iodine deficiency disorder (IDD) still exists in many parts of the world including some areas of the United States. Since it's difficult to accurately measure daily iodine consumption through food sources, iodine deficiency still remains a concern for some vulnerable groups such as pregnant women and children. We'll discuss the challenges associated with identifying and treating iodine deficiency disorders in later chapters.

CHAPTER 3

Iodine Deficiency

Key Points

∝ Your iodine needs change over your lifespan.

∝ According to the World Health Organization (WHO), iodine levels below 100 micrograms per liter (mcg/L) are considered deficient.

∝ Long-term iodine deficiency can lead to thyroid malfunction and cause various health complications.

∝ Certain types of diets can make you more vulnerable to developing iodine deficiency.

As we've learned, iodine deficiency was a common condition in many areas of the world for hundreds of years until universal salt iodization programs were introduced in the early twentieth century. Salt iodization helped to ease high rates of endemic goiter. The United States started salt iodization around 1924, but it wasn't until the 1940s that iodized salt became nationally available for most households. The delay was partly because many people needed convincing that iodine was safe for human use due to its history. But once the majority of US households began using iodized salt, there were improvements in population iodine levels and as a result, endemic goiter rates were significantly reduced.

We've been using iodized salt for many decades now, so iodine deficiency shouldn't be a concern for us anymore, right? Not quite! There is reason to believe there are still some specific groups who may be vulnerable to iodine deficiency, both in the US and around the world.

The majority of iodine you take in (90 percent) is removed through urine within 24 to 48 hours.[33] Your thyroid gland only absorbs a small amount to make thyroid hormones in the correct quantities. Lack of iodine through dietary sources can slowly cause deficiency over time.

There are three dietary reference guidelines to estimate iodine intake developed by the Institute of Medicine's Food and Nutrition Board (a division of the National Academy of Sciences). They include the Recommended Dietary Allowances (RDAs), Estimated Average Requirements (EARs), and Tolerable Upper Intake Levels (ULs). The EAR is used to evaluate the rate of iodine deficiency in the population in a given area, while the RDA is a recommendation of how much iodine an individual should take daily to maintain adequate levels.[34]

According to the World Health Organization, for the general population, iodine deficiency is defined as urine iodine levels below 100 micrograms per liter (µg/L). And, for pregnant women, iodine deficiency is defined as urine iodine levels below 150 µg/L.

Research suggests in order to maintain steady iodine levels in the body for normal thyroid function, we need to take in a minimum amount of iodine daily. This is doable for most people through a normal diet. However, if we continuously get less than this minimum amount of iodine, the thyroid gland cannot produce sufficient amounts of thyroid hormones. Without a proper balance of thyroid hormones, our bodies will start to have problems with metabolism, energy, growth, and development.

33 Elizabeth N. Pearce, Maria Andersson, and Michael B. Zimmermann, "Global Iodine Nutrition: Where Do We Stand In 2013?" *Thyroid* 23, no. 5 (2013): 523–28, doi: 10.1089 /thy.2013.0128.

34 WenYen Juan et al., "Comparison of 2 Methods for Estimating the Prevalences of Inadequate and Excessive Iodine Intakes," *The American Journal of Clinical Nutrition* 104 (2016): 888S–97S, doi: 10.3945/ajcn.115.110346.

Iodine Recommended Daily Allowance (RDA), National Library of Medicine[35]

Population Group or Age	Institute of Medicine Recommended Daily Allowance
Birth to 6 months (acceptable intake)	110 mcg per day
Infant (acceptable intake)	130 mcg per day
Children 1–8 years	90 mcg per day
Children 9–13 years	120 mcg per day
Adolescents (14–18 years)	150 mcg per day
Adults (19 years and older)	150 mcg per day
Pregnant women	220 mcg per day
Breastfeeding women	290 mcg per day

Iodine Recommended Nutrient Intake, World Health Organization[36]

Population Group or Age	World Health Organization Recommended Nutrient Intake
Birth to 5 years	90 mcg per day
Children 6–12 years	120 mcg per day
Adolescents 13 years and older	150 mcg per day
Adults (19 years and older)	150 mcg per day

35 National Institutes of Health (NIH) Office of Dietary Supplements (ODS), "Iodine," last accessed November 30, 2022, https://ods.od.nih.gov/factsheets/Iodine-HealthProfessional.

36 World Health Organization, United Nations Children's Fund & International Council for the Control of Iodine Deficiency Disorders, *Assessment of Iodine Deficiency Disorders and Monitoring Their Elimination*, 3rd ed (Geneva, Switzerland: WHO, 2007).

Iodine Recommended Nutrient Intake, World Health Organization[36]

Population Group or Age	World Health Organization Recommended Nutrient Intake
Pregnant women	250 mcg per day
Breastfeeding women	250 mcg per day

Long-standing iodine deficiency can cause your thyroid gland to malfunction and trigger other health complications; this includes a serious condition known as *thyrotoxicosis*. This is when too much thyroid hormone is circulating in your blood. Thyrotoxicosis typically affects more women than men, and if left untreated can cause serious health problems.

Symptoms of thyrotoxicosis include the following:

∝ menstruation-related (period) changes

∝ sudden weight loss

∝ muscle weakness

∝ mood changes (anxiety, irritability)

∝ shakiness

∝ fast heart rate or irregular heartbeat (arrhythmia)

∝ life-threatening thyroid storm (high fever, fast heartbeat, diarrhea, loss of consciousness), which requires immediate emergency medical attention

Data Highlights

Data from the National Health and Nutrition Examination Surveys (NHANES[37]—a program of the Centers for Disease Control and

---

37 NHANES nutrition surveys are conducted annually. Scientific studies continue to examine U.S. population level nutritional status based on the NHANES surveys for different time periods. NHANES-based studies cited in this book list studies of different years for different nutritional status, including iodine.

Prevention) from 2005 to 2010 show there have been declines in estimated population iodine levels in recent years in the United States. Reduced iodine levels among vulnerable groups are especially notable.[38] According to these data, urine iodine levels have been decreasing among various vulnerable groups in the US.

Geographically, the data show California had the lowest average urine iodine levels at 107 µg/L. Pennsylvania had an average level of 125 µg/L, Wisconsin had 145 µg/L, New York had 150 µg/L, and Utah had 190 µg/L. South Dakota and Minnesota both had levels of 205 µg/L, and North Carolina had an average level of 217 µg/L.[39] It's difficult to know the exact cause of these variances in iodine levels in different states, but individual dietary differences, soil, and other environmental factors may all play a role. We'll discuss this in more detail in later chapters.

There were also differences among various racial/ethnic groups. The NHANES study found the average urine iodine levels among non-Hispanic Blacks was 131 µg/L, which was comparatively much lower than other racial/ethnic groups, such as non-Hispanic whites, with an average level of 147 µg/L, and Hispanics, who had an average level of 148 µg/L.[40] One hypothesis potentially accounting for these differences may be the dietary influences of different racial/ethnic groups. We'll discuss this a bit later on.

So, what do all these data mean exactly? In short, they mean iodine deficiency is still a concern in the US. Although we've come a long way in correcting population-level iodine deficiency, and we have reduced occurrences of endemic goiter, recent nutrition data show pregnant women, infants, and those on a vegan diet may be

38 Kathleen L. Caldwell et al., "Iodine Status in Pregnant Women in the National Children's Study and in U.S. Women," *Thyroid* 23, no. 8 (2013): 927–37, doi: 10.1089/thy .2013.0012.

39 Kathleen L. Caldwell et al., "Iodine Status."

40 Kathleen L. Caldwell et al., "Iodine Status."

vulnerable to iodine deficiency. Let's take a look at some of the specific potential health impacts of iodine deficiency.

Health Effects Linked to Iodine Deficiency

Age Group	Conditions
Pregnant Women	Hypothyroidism, miscarriage, anemia, stillbirth, preeclampsia, pre-term birth, vulnerability to nuclear radiation exposure
Fetal	Congenital hypothyroidism, impaired mental and physical development, deafness, risk of perinatal death, vulnerability to nuclear radiation exposure
Newborn	Hypothyroidism, impaired physical and mental development, increased risk of infant death
Children and Adolescents	Goiter, impaired physical and brain development, learning disabilities, poor educational achievement, compromised intellectual growth, vulnerability to nuclear radiation exposure
Adults	Goiter, hypothyroidism, impaired mental development, increased risk of thyroid cancer from radiation exposure, infertility in females, hormonal irregularities in males and females, coronary artery disease, dyslipidemia (high blood lipids), vulnerability to nuclear radiation exposure

Coronary Artery Disease

In the United States, coronary artery disease (CAD) is the most common form of heart disease. It occurs when the major arteries supplying blood to the heart are blocked or impaired. This can happen from an inflammation of or a narrowing of arteries because of cholesterol buildup. A 2017 study based on the NHANES 2007–2012 nutrition survey found that those with low urine iodine levels had a higher risk of coronary artery disease.[41] But the exact link is still unclear. For example, does having low iodine levels directly cause coronary artery disease or does it increase the risks for CAD? Scientists still aren't sure. However, it's an important finding that certainly needs further investigation.

Studies have also shown obesity, particularly in women, can cause alterations in metabolism and lead to mineral imbalances in the body. This is significant since metabolic disorders can cause other chronic (long-standing) health conditions such as diabetes, heart disease, non-alcoholic fatty liver disease, and cancer.[42] According to the WHO and the CDC, having a body mass index (BMI) above 25 kg/m^2 is considered being overweight, and a BMI above 30 kg/m^2 is considered obese. According to data from WHO, in 2016 nearly 2 billion adults worldwide were overweight and of this group, 650 million were considered obese.

Obesity can lead to less absorption of minerals, including lower magnesium, selenium, iodine, and zinc levels, and higher levels of copper. Studies have shown obesity can cause iodine deficiency and poor iodine absorption.[43] However, more studies are needed to better understand the role of obesity in iodine absorption and the exact cause of iodine deficiency.

41 H. V. Tran, N. Erskine et al., "Is Low Iodine a Risk Factor for Cardiovascular Disease in Americans Without Thyroid Dysfunction? Findings from NHANES," *Nutrition, Metabolism and Cardiovascular Diseases* 27, no. 7 (2017): 651–56.

42 W. Banach et al., "The Association Between Excess Body Mass and Disturbances in Somatic Mineral Levels," *International Journal of Molecular Sciences* 21, no. 19 (2013): 7306, doi: 10.3390/ijms21197306.

43 H. V. Tran et al., "Is Low Iodine a Risk Factor for Cardiovascular Disease in Americans Without Thyroid Dysfunction? Findings from NHANES," *Nutrition Metabolism and Cardiovascular Diseases* 7 (2017): 651–656, doi: 10.1016/j.numecd.2017.06.001; Albert Lecube, "Iodine Deficiency Is Higher in Morbid Obesity in Comparison with Late After Bariatric Surgery and Non-Obese Women," *Obesity Surgery* 25, no. 1 (2015): 85–9, doi: 10.1007/s11695-014-1313-z.

Dyslipidemia

Dyslipidemia indicates abnormal levels of certain kinds of lipids (fats) in your blood. Generally, dyslipidemia can mean your total cholesterol levels, triglycerides, or low-density lipoproteins (LDL) levels are too high. But it may also mean your high-density lipoprotein (HDL) levels are too low or a combination of these imbalances. LDL is referred to as the "bad" cholesterol because it can build up in the arteries causing narrowing or blockages, which can lead to CAD.

On the other hand, HDL is referred to as "good" cholesterol because it helps to remove LDL from the blood. Triglycerides are fats you take in through calories you consume, which, when not used for energy, are stored in fat cells in the body. In the long term, when you eat more calories than you burn, you may have increased triglyceride levels, which can raise your risk of heart-related problems such as heart attack or stroke. There are many causes for dyslipidemia, including family history and lifestyle factors.

A 2016 study based on the 2007–2012 NHANES nutrition survey data compared two groups of adults 20 years or older who either had low or normal iodine levels.[44] The study found those individuals with low iodine levels had abnormal cholesterol levels compared with those with higher iodine levels. In particular, women over 60 years of age had higher total cholesterol and LDL and other lipid levels. And those who were in the upper 10 percentile of urine iodine levels had normal cholesterol ranges.

Other studies have found iodine levels greater than 100 μg/L had a beneficial effect on cholesterol levels, compared with having low iodine levels. An older 1995 study also found that giving iodine supplements for six months improved lipid levels. However, more research is needed to understand the connections between iodine

---

44 K. Lee, D. Shin. and W. Song, "Low Urinary Iodine Concentrations Associated with Dyslipidemia in US Adults," *Nutrients* 8, no. 3 (2016): 171.

levels and lipid abnormalities.[45] You shouldn't supplement iodine on your own if you have high cholesterol without consulting your doctor. This is because scientists still don't know the exact link between iodine deficiency and lipid levels. And there may be other reasons for lipid imbalances.

However, one scientific theory is that there may be a connection between low iodine levels and high cholesterol levels from poor functioning of the thyroid gland. Since thyroid hormones help regulate metabolism in the body, with a low-functioning thyroid, hypothyroidism may cause increased body weight, abnormal cholesterol levels, and reduced breakdown of fats. Hypothyroidism also increases the risk of heart disease and elevated cholesterol.

Iodine deficiency has also been associated with an increase in circulating thyroid-stimulating hormone (TSH). This is a reaction by the body that allows more iodine to be taken up in the blood to regulate thyroid hormones. Research indicates elevated TSH may increase the risk for abnormal lipid levels.

Low iodine levels may contribute to metabolic changes and trigger shifts in TSH levels, which cause a cascade of related health effects including increased LDL levels. This is why it's crucial to understand the connections between low iodine levels and certain health disorders that may be corrected through iodine balancing.

There is still much more to learn about iodine's possible protective role in health and disease.

---

45 Dandan Wang et al., "Associations Between Water Iodine Concentration and the Prevalence of Dyslipidemia in Chinese Adults: A Cross-Sectional Study," *Ecotoxicology Environmental Safety* 208 (2021): 11682, doi: 10.1016/j.ecoenv.2020.111682; G. Rönnefarth et al., "Euthyroid Goiter in Puberty—A Harmless Illness?" *Klinische Padiatre* 208, no. 2 (1996): 77–82, doi: 10.1055/s-2008-1043999; Kyung Won Lee, Dayeon Shin, and Won O. Song, "Low Urinary Iodine Concentrations Associated with Dyslipidemia in US Adults," *Nutrients* 8, no. 3 (2016): 171, doi: 10.3390/nu8030171.

Goiter

While there are different causes and types of goiter, one of the most common causes is iodine deficiency. As noted earlier, *endemic goiter* refers to goiter caused by iodine deficiency from inadequate iodine in food or water sources in a given region.[46] While incidences of serious endemic goiter have diminished, endemic goiter continues to occur in many parts of the world with poor environmental iodine conditions (soil and water).

Goiter may involve growth of the entire thyroid gland, or it might be due to abnormal cell growth that causes nodules or lumps to form in the thyroid gland. Endemic goiter is more common in females than males, and among adolescents and pregnant women. Recall that iodine needs are higher during certain periods of life such as during pregnancy.

Children with endemic goiter typically have swelling of the thyroid gland, with or without changes in thyroid hormone production. However, adults generally have nodular forms of goiter. Diagnosis typically involves determining the cause of goiter, among them iodine deficiency, exposure to goitrogens (explained on page 52), autoimmune-related thyroid conditions, nodular goiter, infection, inflammation, cyst, and cancer.

Goiters may either cause shifts in thyroid hormone production (up or down), or in mild cases, there may be no changes in thyroid function. The treatment for goiter also depends on the type and size of the goiter, and on other factors involved such as any health complications.

Generally, with mild cases, there are no symptoms with goiter other than an outward swelling at the bottom of the front of the neck

---

46 Gregory A. Brent and Anthony P. Weetman, "Chapter 13–Hypothyroidism and Thyroiditis," *Williams Textbook of Endocrinology*, 13th ed. (2016): 416–18, doi: 10.1016 /B978-0-323-29738-7.00013-7.

if there is no hypothyroidism. In fact, small growths can often go undetected until another health concern leads to a diagnosis.

In cases of mild or moderate iodine deficiency, the thyroid gland may become enlarged to increase the uptake of iodine to provide the body with enough thyroid hormones as an adjustment. However, with serious iodine deficiency, a large goiter can obstruct the trachea and create difficulties with breathing and speech. And nodular goiter can cause hemorrhaging, pain, and swelling. Long term, it can also lead to damage to the nerves of the larynx (voice box).

Other effects may include difficulty swallowing, a cough, and a hoarse voice. Goiter can also be caused by exposure to goitrogens, which are natural or chemical compounds that can interfere with normal thyroid function and cause a swelling of the thyroid gland as a reaction. Generally, exposure to low levels of goitrogens doesn't have much of an impact.. But you may be particularly sensitive to goitrogens if your iodine levels are already low, or if you're exposed to goitrogenic substances for long periods of time.

Goitrogens can lower the amount of iodine your thyroid gland can take up, lower the amount of thyroid-stimulating hormone (TSH) and T4 produced by the thyroid gland, and cause thyroid gland enlargement.

There are three main categories of food-based goitrogens. They include the following:

∝ flavonoids
∝ thiocyanates
∝ goitrins

Flavonoid compounds are found naturally in many fruits, vegetables, and plants. Research has shown flavonoids have many healthful properties such as anti-inflammatory and antioxidant effects. Examples of natural products rich in flavonoids include berries, grapefruit, lemons, green tea, lettuce, kale, grapes, red peppers, celery, and red wine.

While flavonoid compounds have many health benefits, taking too many of some of these compounds can interfere with thyroid function. This is especially true if you're iodine deficient or have thyroid-related conditions.

Thiocyanates can block the amount of iodide going into the thyroid follicular cells. This can lower the amount of thyroxine made by the thyroid gland. This can cause thryoid imbalances in people who are more susceptible to shifts in iodine levels. Some plant-based sources of thiocyanate include yam, sweet potato, cassava, and corn. In some regions of Africa, increased use of cassava along with selenium deficiency and inconsistent iodine supplementation has led to greater degrees of endemic goiter and other related thyroid conditions.

Many plants have goitrogenic properties and can interfere with thyroid function. While they have beneficial effects, people with thyroid problems, or those who may have serious iodine deficiency, may experience thyroid-related problems with heavy consumption.

Some examples of goitrins include kale, brussels sprouts, mustard greens, and cabbage. Cooking these vegetables can be helpful in reducing their goitrogenic effects. If you have an existing thyroid condition or are iodine deficient, talk with your doctor about goitrogenic foods.

Examples of Goitrogens[47]

Categories	Examples
Foods	Broccoli, cabbage, cauliflower, kale, turnips, soy, millet, lima beans, cassava, sweet potato, collard greens, berries, teas, and more

47 W. Banach et al., "The Association Between Excess Body Mass and Disturbances in Somatic Mineral Levels."

Examples of Goitrogens[47]

Categories	Examples
Chemical Compounds	Polyhalogenated hydrocarbons, polybrominated (PBB) and polychlorinated (PCB) biphenyls (added to plastics such as televisions, computer monitors, upholstery, rugs, plastic foam, etc.), pesticides (chlorobenziate, DDT, lindane, dioxin), and more
Nutrient Deficiencies	Iron, selenium, and vitamin A deficiencies can interfere with normal thyroid function

If you have a lump at the lower part of the front of your neck or have symptoms of goiter, make an appointment to see a doctor for a diagnosis. They'll check your thyroid gland and how it's functioning. Your doctor may order blood tests and other tests such as an ultrasound, a computed tomography (CT) scan, a biopsy, or a urine iodine test. They'll also discuss your diet and other nutritional factors that may interfere with thyroid function.

The treatment for goiter depends on the condition's severity, cause, and options available. Treatment may include surgery if the goiter is obstructing breathing.

For mild goiter caused by iodine deficiency, correcting iodine levels may be sufficient to improve goiter and restore normal thyroid function. Your doctor will go over all the treatment options based on your individual health needs.

We'll discuss the various types of iodine treatments available along with good dietary sources of iodine later in the book.

Hypothyroidism

Hypothyroidism refers to a condition in which the thyroid gland is underactive and doesn't make enough thyroid hormones. As mentioned, thyroid hormones help regulate many vital body functions such as digestion, temperature regulation, heart rate, energy levels, and much more.

There are many different causes for hypothyroidism, but globally, iodine deficiency is still considered the most common cause of hypothyroidism in adults.[48] Environmental factors such as soil, water, and nutrition all play a role. The condition is more common in women than men. If you have a history of iodine deficiency or thyroid-related conditions, such as hypothyroidism or hyperthyroidism, your body is more prone to iodine-related thyroid conditions.

Other causes of hypothyroidism include the following:

- radiation therapy
- radioactive iodine treatment
- thyroid surgery
- Hashimoto's thyroiditis
- certain medications
- problems with the pituitary gland
- pregnancy (some women may develop hypothyroidism after pregnancy called *postpartum thyroiditis*)

Hashimoto's thyroiditis is also called *chronic autoimmune lymphocytic thyroiditis*. It is the most common cause of an underactive thyroid in the United States. It is an autoimmune condition in which your body's own white blood cells and antibodies attack the cells of your thyroid gland, damaging thyroid function.

Scientists don't know the exact cause of Hashimoto's thyroiditis but believe genetic factors may play a role. For example, if you have a family history of certain autoimmune disorders (Graves' disease, type 1 diabetes, Addison's disease, lupus, rheumatoid arthritis), you may have a higher risk of developing the condition.

---

48 Amir Babiker et al., "The Role of Micronutrients in Thyroid Dysfunction," *Sudanese Journal of Paediatrics* 20, no. 1 (2020): 13–19, doi: 10.24911/SJP.106-1587138942.

Hypothyroidism may also be caused by radiation treatment for certain types of cancers, radioactive iodine treatment for hyperthyroidism (overactive thyroid), surgery to remove the thyroid gland, or certain medications (amiodarone, lithium, stavudine, and others). Your doctor can provide more details about all the possible causes of hypothyroidism.

Symptoms of hypothyroidism include the following:

- excessive tiredness
- brittle nails
- constipation
- depression
- headaches
- slowed heart rate
- high cholesterol
- goiter
- problems with learning or memory
- dry skin
- cold hands and feet
- hair loss
- muscle weakness
- fertility issues, menstrual irregularity, pregnancy problems in women
- joint stiffness
- puffy face
- weight gain
- slow growth in children

Since thyroid disorders can occur for many different reasons, you may need several different tests to diagnose the cause of hypothyroidism.

If you have symptoms of an underactive thyroid, such as neck swelling, slow heart rate, or other physical signs, your doctor will order certain blood tests to check your thyroid function.

One test is a thyroid-stimulating hormone (TSH) test. This determines how much TSH your pituitary gland is making. The normal range of TSH is between 0.4 to 4.0 milli-international units per liter if you're not on thyroid treatment. If the TSH level is high, it means you have an underactive thyroid gland. Your pituitary gland is making more TSH to activate the thyroid gland to make more thyroid hormones. Remember the negative feedback loop we discussed on page 16? Basically, the pituitary gland creates TSH to urge the thyroid gland to make thyroid hormones. Too much or too little TSH and your thyroid gland function is affected.

If your TSH levels are low, this means you have an overactive (hyperthyroid) condition. Your pituitary gland is making less TSH because your thyroid gland is making too much thyroid hormone.

Other tests to check your thyroid function include the thyroxine (T4) test. As we discussed in chapter 1, T4 is a thyroid hormone produced by the thyroid gland. If your T4 level is low and your TSH is high, you may be hypothyroid. If your T4 level is normal, your doctor may check your triiodothyronine (T3) level. If your T3 level is low, you may have hypothyroidism.

Keep in mind, since there are several causes of hypothyroidism depending on your individual factors, your doctor may check your iodine levels and do other tests they feel are appropriate to diagnose the cause of your thyroid condition.

If your hypothyroidism is related to iodine deficiency, your doctor will discuss available treatments including nutrition and diet that can impact your thyroid function. They may talk with you about avoiding or limiting goitrogenic foods such as soy products, which can interfere with thyroid function if you're seriously iodine deficient.

If you're pregnant or planning to become pregnant, having balanced iodine levels for a properly functioning thyroid gland is important for a normal pregnancy and for the health of your baby.

Risks of hypothyroidism during pregnancy include the following:

- miscarriage
- anemia
- stillbirth
- preeclampsia
- pre-term birth
- low birth weight
- birth defects
- problems with fetal brain development

Tell your doctor if you have a history of thyroid-related disorders or iodine deficiency. They may check your thyroid function and monitor you during your pregnancy and after delivery for any thyroid-related problems.

Impaired Brain and Physical Development

Iodine is an essential micronutrient that's a key component of thyroid hormone necessary for normal brain and physical development, particularly during fetal development and early infancy. Iodine deficiency is the most common preventable cause of impaired brain development.

Micronutrients support normal pregnancy and growth of a fetus. An unborn baby's thyroid gland doesn't start making thyroid hormones until the second trimester of pregnancy (around 20 weeks' gestation). A mother's free T4 thyroid hormone contributes to the total thyroid hormone levels of an unborn baby and of a newborn.[49] This is why having balanced iodine levels during pregnancy is crucial for normal fetal and infant development.

A newborn experiences a sharp increase in thyroid-stimulating hormone (TSH) shortly after birth (30–60 minutes), which helps stimulate the thyroid gland to make T4 and T3. Infants make three times the amount of T4 as do adults, but both T4 and T3 levels start to drop off slowly in the first few days after birth. Levels of thyroid hormones continue to slowly drop during infancy and childhood. But babies are born with very little stored iodine and rely on breast milk or infant formula to meet their iodine needs to continue making T4.

This is why during pregnancy a woman's iodine needs increase to support pregnancy and a developing baby. Serious iodine deficiency during pregnancy may cause low-functioning thyroid and hypothy-

---

49 Sheila A. Skeaff, "Iodine Deficiency in Pregnancy: The Effect on Neurodevelopment in the Child," *Nutrients* 3, no. 2 (2011): 265–73, doi: 10.3390/nu3020265.

roidism for both the mother and unborn baby with compromised health outcomes for both. Scientists are also learning more about the effects of mild to moderate iodine deficiency on fetal brain and physical development.

Changes in thyroid function are common in women shortly after delivery, and many women experience hypo- or hyperthyroidism during this time compared with before or during pregnancy. The incidence of autoimmune thyroiditis (thyroid gland inflammation) after delivery is around 5 percent, and it usually happens between one and four months after delivery. It's typically more common in women who already had mild thyroiditis prior to pregnancy. This thyroiditis then might worsen after delivery.

The pathway of the condition involves having temporary thyro-toxicosis, which turns into temporary hypothyroidism, followed by a return to normal thyroid function (euthyroid). Normal thyroid function typically returns at the end of the first year after delivery unless there is an existing thyroid disorder complicating thyroid recovery.

Although iodine deficiency is known to increase the risk for thyroid disorders, studies so far haven't proven iodine deficiency in pregnancy causes thyroiditis post-delivery. However, it has not been ruled out as a possible contributing cause of thyroid disorder. More research is needed to understand the impact of various iodine levels on pregnancy and post-delivery, particularly since evidence indicates many women are mildly iodine deficient during pregnancy.

According to WHO, children are considered to be mildly iodine deficient with urine iodine concentration levels between 50 and 99 µg/L. With the advent of salt iodization, much of the devel-oping world is iodine sufficient. But because salt iodization is not mandated in most countries, millions of people around the world are at risk for mild or moderate iodine deficiency. In fact, studies show an estimated 350 million people in Europe do not have access to iodized salt and are at risk of mild to moderate iodine deficiency.[50]

There is an urgent need for better designed studies to learn what effects (if any) mild or moderate iodine deficiency has on pregnant and lactating women and on the development of unborn babies and infants. A 2020 study of pregnant women in Bangkok, Thailand, with mild iodine deficiency who received daily iodine supplements found there was no effect on child development and a mildly negative effect on thyroid hormone levels in the mothers.[51]

There is a lack of information on the safety and effectiveness of iodine supplementation in mild or moderate iodine deficiency. This is important since nutritional survey data on women in many regions of the world, including the United States, have shown many women have mild or moderate iodine deficiency. Does the body compensate for mild deficiency during pregnancy? What about moderate deficiency? Are there any long-term child development consequences?

So far, the answers to these questions are still unclear. Some studies indicate there may be brain and physical development impairments in children when mothers have moderate iodine deficiency.[52] But more conclusive evidence, including other factors that may contribute to negative effects, is needed. Currently, there is also a lack of consensus among public health experts on appro-

50 World Health Organization, "Urinary Iodine Concentrations for Determining Iodine Status in Populations. Vitamin and Mineral Nutrition Information System," 2013, www.who.int/nutrition/vmnis/indicators/urinaryiodine; Elizabeth N. Peace et al., "Consequences of Iodine Deficiency and Excess in Pregnant Women: An Overview of Current Knowns and Unknowns," *American Journal of Clinical Nutrition* (2016): 918S–23S, doi: 10.3945/ajcn.115.110429.

51 Nicole J. E. Verhagen et al., "Iodine Supplementation in Mildly Iodine-Deficient Pregnant Women Does Not Improve Maternal Thyroid Function or Child Development: A Secondary Analysis of a Randomized Controlled Trial," *Frontiers in Endocrinology* (October 6, 2020): 11:572984, doi: 10.3389/fendo.2020.572984.

52 F. Delange, "Iodine Deficiency as a Cause of Brain Damage," *Postgraduate Medical Journal* 77 (2001): 217–20, doi: 10.1136/pmj.77.906.217.

priate dosing for iodine supplementation and safe upper limits for pregnant and lactating women who are deficient.

Scientists are also exploring what deficiencies in related micronutrients, such as selenium and iron along with iodine, have on pregnancy and fetal development. This is an area that needs more research because some studies have shown there is a link between low iron levels, higher TSH levels, and lower T4 levels in regions where there is mild iodine deficiency. Iron and selenium are also important micronutrients for a healthy pregnancy and normal fetal growth and development.

Currently, to prevent pregnancy-related iodine deficiency, the International Federation of Gynecology and Obstetrics recommends using iodized salt, but where there is limited access to iodized salt, they recommend supplementing iodine at 250 µg per day.[53]

Just as severely low iodine levels during pregnancy are harmful for both mothers and babies, too much iodine (excess iodine) is also harmful and can affect proper thyroid function. Excess iodine may trigger thyroid hormone imbalances in pregnant women and cause thyroid-related autoimmune conditions.

Thyroid Cancer

Thyroid cancer, specifically papillary thyroid cancer (PTC) and follicular thyroid cancer (FTC), is the most common form of endocrine-related cancer worldwide.[54] Although the exact cause of different types of thyroid cancers is unknown, iodine deficiency is considered a risk factor for certain thyroid cancers, particularly FTC.

---

53 Alison D. Gernand et al., "Micronutrient Deficiencies in Pregnancy Worldwide: Health Effects and Prevention," *Nature Review Endocrinology* 12, no. 5 (2016): 274–89, doi: 10.1038/nrendo.2016.37.

54 Lulu L. Sakafu et al., "Thyroid Cancer and Iodine Deficiency Status: A 10-Year Review at a Single Cancer Center in Tanzania," *OTO Open* 2, no. 2 (2018), doi: 10.1177 /2473974X18777238.

Research has shown long-standing, serious iodine deficiency causes overstimulation of TSH and thyroid gland malfunction. This causes abnormal changes in the thyroid gland. Access to iodized salt and consuming adequate iodine through diet are important measures to maintain thyroid hormone balance.

There may not be any early signs or symptoms of thyroid cancer because it grows slowly. Most people are diagnosed when they or their doctor notice a neck nodule.

Symptoms may include the following:

- nodule in the neck
- trouble breathing or swallowing
- painful swallowing
- fever
- hoarse voice
- weight loss

Breast Cancer

There is a lack of definitive evidence for any link between iodine deficiency and breast cancer. Iodine is found in breast tissue and helps encourage normal tissue development. Iodine also has antioxidant effects and offers protective effects on breast tissue. More research is needed to better understand the possible role of iodine for breast health.

Special Dietary Considerations

Ethno-cultural factors influence dietary choices worldwide and can certainly impact nutrition levels including the micronutrient iodine. For example, studies have shown vegans have a higher risk for iodine deficiency due to their dietary preferences.[55]

---

55 Angela M. Leung et al., "Iodine Status and Thyroid Function of Boston-Area Vegetarians and Vegans," *Journal of Clinical Endocrinology* 96, no. 8 (2011): E1303–7,

This is primarily because traditional dairy products (based on cow's milk), and products such as seafood, eggs, and bread have higher amounts of iodine than other types of foods such as vegetables. Eliminating iodine rich sources of food and substituting primarily plant-based food sources can increase the risk for low iodine levels because fruits and vegetables have insignificant amounts of iodine.

If you follow specific dietary practices, it's important to be aware of causes and consequences of long-term iodine deficiency. You may need to supplement iodine in your diet to make sure you don't develop thyroid problems.

If you do follow a special diet, it may be helpful to locate a culturally competent dietitian or nutritionist who can work with you to develop food resources of iodine-rich foods. A culturally relevant nutritional guide incorporates cultural influences for your diet and can provide recommendations that respect your choices based on your ethnicity, culture, or individual beliefs.

This may be particularly impactful if you're pregnant and follow a vegan diet. Collaborating with a culturally sensitive dietitian can help you communicate your dietary needs effectively to develop goals for maintaining nutritional balance, including iodine levels.

Understanding Health Disparities

You've likely been hearing a lot about health disparities in the media lately as a result of the Covid-19 pandemic. The ongoing pandemic has changed the world in many fundamental ways. It has certainly heightened awareness about our reliance on the healthcare system in the communities where we live. Can we count on it to take care of us? What is the quality of care we'll receive? What factors affect

doi: 10.1210/jc.2011-0256.

our care? Does the type of care we receive depend on our race, ethnicity, income, gender? That seems unthinkable, right?

If you've never thought about these questions, you likely haven't been touched by health disparities. But they do exist and impact many millions of people and the care they receive every day. Health disparities are avoidable inequalities associated with a health condition, an injury, or the ability of certain groups to achieve optimal health due to lack of resources and socioeconomic factors.

Data have shown that health disparities disproportionately impact certain underrepresented racial, ethnic, and socioeconomically disadvantaged groups. And these populations experience worse outcomes from preventable diseases, injuries, and other medical concerns. These effects can last for multiple generations. For example, disparities affecting a pregnant mother may also affect her baby, perpetuating poor outcomes for years.

Although health disparities have been a part of population-level statistics for generations, their impact has not been well documented until recently, particularly for some groups. However, since the pandemic began, public health organizations, policy-focused organizations, and other affected groups have been actively raising awareness and promoting inclusiveness to improve health equity.

Poor representation of diverse racial/ethnic groups in scientific research studies for health conditions has negatively affected individual and community wellness, and resource allocation—which can last for years.

This is because some of these groups were not included in disease metrics, creating knowledge gaps. But scientists are beginning to acknowledge that race, ethnicity, and socio-environmental-related factors play an important role in disease prevalence, progression, and outcomes. And inclusion of broad population representation that makes up a community's ethnic and racial diversity is crucial to understanding the public health needs of the community.

What Contributes to Health Disparities?

Research shows causes of health disparities are complex and many factors are involved. They include discrimination, trauma, cultural bias, and other socio-environmental issues, such as housing, employment, pollution, education, income, and resource availability. Continued unequal access to the resources necessary to improve the quality of life also contributes to health disparities.

How Can Health Disparities Be Improved?

Changes to the social determinants of health (SDOH) can help lower risks associated with health disparities. SDOH are socio-environmental conditions in places people live, learn, work, and socialize that affect their quality of life and health. Public health programs and partnerships with community stakeholders to improve healthcare access; health literacy (understanding health information); and wellness initiatives to expand access to affordable, healthy foods and lifestyle choices can all make a difference.

Globally, iodine deficiency disproportionately impacts socioeconomically disadvantaged communities. Factors such as where someone lives and their access to nutritious foods impacts health. This includes lack of access to iodized salt, which can increase the risk of iodine deficiency.

Disparities in Disease Prevalence: Who's at Risk for Iodine Deficiency?

Since the discovery of iodine's role in thyroid health became known, rates of endemic goiter and severe iodine deficiency have been reduced considerably around the world. This is largely due to access to and use of iodized salt in a majority of households. We've known that iodine deficiency is a preventable condition for more than a hundred years, so why are there still millions at risk for this condition? The health disparities described in the preceding section are a primary reason.

Severe iodine deficiency still exists in communities where people live in poor environmental conditions. They don't have access to nutritious food sources because of the aforementioned social determinants of health where they live, or they don't have access to iodized salt. Serious iodine deficiency is still common in parts of Africa, Asia, Eastern Europe, and the eastern Mediterranean regions.[56]

There are other areas of the world experiencing mild to moderate iodine deficiency for various reasons. They include countries such as Iraq, Finland, Norway, Russia, Lebanon, Israel, Italy, and others.[57] In addition, some specific vulnerable groups, such as those on restrictive diets and those living in areas where the soil and water have been depleted of iodine, are also susceptible to iodine deficiency.

---

56 Iwona Krela-Kaźmierczak et al., "Is There an Ideal Diet to Protect Against Iodine Deficiency?" *Nutrients* 13, no. 2 (2020): 513, doi: 10.3390/nu13020513.

57 Cinzia Giordano et al., "Endemic Goiter and Iodine Prophylaxis in Calabria, a Region of Southern Italy: Past and Present," *Nutrients* 11, no. 10 (2019): 2428, doi: 10.3390/nu11102428.

Mild iodine deficiency exists all over the world. According to the World Health Organization, more than 50 million people have brain impairment linked to iodine deficiency.[58] Iodine deficiency has long-term implications because research has shown serious iodine deficiency during early stages of brain development can lower intelligence quotient (IQ) by as much as 15 points.

Measuring iodine levels for various age groups is unreliable because it's difficult to get accurate results, and this can create challenges in defining who needs iodine supplements or dietary changes. The most vulnerable groups at risk for iodine deficiency are those who need higher amounts to support normal thyroid hormone function during certain periods of growth, and those without access to robust nutritional resources.

Exposure to certain environmental factors can also increase the risk of iodine deficiency due to blocking of iodine uptake by the body. For example, research has shown that contact with certain toxins such as nitrate, perchlorate, and thiocyanate can block iodine from being absorbed by the thyroid gland and the intestine. These products are readily found in the environment, causing common human exposure through water and food sources. For example, thiocyanate is found in milk and vegetables.[59]

A Canadian study found that diet (low dairy and iodized salt intake), being vegan or vegetarian, environmental conditions (where people live), and smoking were associated with higher risks for iodine deficiency.[60]

---

58 World Health Organization, "Nutrition: Effects of Iodine Deficiency," May 2013, https://www.who.int/news-room/questions-and-answers/item/nutrition-effects-of-iodine-deficiency.

59 N. Mervish, A. Pajak, et al., "Thyroid Antagonists (Perchlorate, Thiocyanate, and Nitrate) and Childhood Growth in a Longitudinal Study of U.S. Girls," *Environmental Health Perspectives* 124, no. 4 (2016): 542–49.

60 Gerhard Eisenbrand and Heinz-Peter Gelbke, "Assessing the Potential Impact on the Thyroid Axis of Environmentally Relevant Food Constituents/Contaminants in Humans," *Archives of Toxicology* 90, 2016: 1841–57, doi: 10.1007/s00204-016-1735 -6; Sun Y. Lee et al., "Urinary Iodine, Perchlorate, and Thiocyanate Concentrations in

Since a developing unborn baby relies solely on a mother's thyroid hormones in early pregnancy, it's important for women of child-bearing age to have adequate iodine levels. This is particularly significant since 40 percent of pregnancies are unplanned.[61]

Vulnerable groups include the following:

- pregnant women
- breastfeeding women
- unborn babies
- newborns and infants
- those following special diets

We'll get into more detail about the iodine content of common foods in chapter 7. For now, it's important to highlight that dairy products, eggs, seafood, and bread have high amounts of iodine. If you avoid or eliminate high iodine food categories such as dairy, eggs, seafood, and bread from your diet, you may be at increased risk for long-term iodine deficiency. This is particularly true if other dietary nutritional replacements are not substituted to compensate for dietary restrictions.

In the United States, a majority of iodine intake comes from dairy products. It is estimated to be around 60–70 percent of iodine intake for 6- to 12-year-olds, and nearly 50 percent of intake for adults. Some other sources include iodized salt, water, and supplements, which comprise around 10–20 percent of total intake.

U.S. Lactating Women," *Thyroid* 27, no. 12 (2017): 1574–81, doi: 10.1089/thy.2017.0158; Craig Steinmaus et al., "Combined Effects of Perchlorate, Thiocyanate, and Iodine on Thyroid Function in the National Health and Nutrition Examination Survey 2007–08," *Environmental Research, no.* 123 (2013): 17–24, doi: 10.1016/j.envres.2013.01.005; Stellena Mathiaparanam et al., "The Prevalence and Risk Factors Associated with Iodine Deficiency in Canadian Adults," *Nutrients* 14, no. 13 (2022): 2570, doi: 10.3390/nu14132570.

61 Kirsten A. Herrick, "Iodine Status and Consumption of Key Iodine Sources in the U.S. Population with Special Attention to Reproductive Age Women," *Nutrients* 10, no. 7 (2018): E874, doi: 10.3390/nu10070874.

However, it's difficult to accurately predict iodine levels in food sources since other factors such as the type of animal feed, geographic location, or presence of goitrogens in feed can cause shifts in levels.

Iodine Status and Consumption of Key Iodine Sources in the US Population with Special Attention to Reproductive-Age Women (NHANES 2011–2014)[62]

Racial/Ethnic Group*	Asian	Black	Hispanic	White
Urine iodine level	81 µg/L	124 µg/L	133 µg/L	106 µg/L
Dairy consumption	119 grams	113 grams	154 grams	162 grams
Grain consumption	388 grams	308 grams	343 grams	293 grams
Soy consumption (goitrogen that may block iodine uptake)	18 grams	1 gram	9 grams	8 grams

*Participants were non-pregnant, non-lactating women, 15–44 years.

The study found that certain Asian groups had higher consumption of soy products and seaweed, while Black Americans had lower dairy consumption. Asian women were found to be mildly iodine deficient based on urine iodine levels.

It's still not clear how much diet, race, or other individual genetic factors contribute to low iodine levels among certain racial/ethnic groups. Future studies that examine the role of ethno-cultural and other dietary and socio-environmental considerations linked to iodine deficiency will be valuable in shaping iodine level requirement recommendations for different population groups.

A majority of US households is thought to be iodine sufficient. Further, a majority (70 percent) of salt intake in the United

---

62 Kirsten A. Herrick, "Iodine Status."

States comes from foods prepared outside the home (restaurant, commercial), which are not necessarily made with iodized salt.[63] And in only around 53 percent of households, table salt is iodized.[64] Interestingly, people who used less salt had higher urine iodine levels. Since the US nutrition survey data (NHANES) don't capture the types of salt consumed (iodized vs. non-iodized) it's difficult to tell how salt consumption contributes to iodine levels. But certainly, this is an important area to understand for those on salt-restrictive diets due to health reasons such as high blood pressure.

Researchers also need to better understand how diet affects certain groups who require higher amounts of iodine, and what factors may contribute to low iodine levels in these groups. Learning the effects of dietary patterns for specific racial/ethnic groups may help to ensure balanced iodine levels, especially for vulnerable groups.

Further research is needed to factor differences in iodine intake based on ethno-cultural dietary habits and food consumption that have not been well documented in research studies so far.

Signs and Symptoms of Iodine Deficiency

Your iodine requirements depend on your age, and also change at different stages of your life. If you have normal iodine levels, only 10 percent of the iodine you take in through diet is retained by the thyroid gland; the rest is removed through urine. However, in people with long-lasting iodine deficiency, the thyroid gland will try to capture nearly 80 percent of the iodine circulating in the blood. This is to compensate for low iodine levels to allow the thyroid gland to

---

63 Lisa J. Harnack, "Sources of Sodium in US Adults from 3 Geographic Regions," *Circulation* 135 (2017): 1775–83, doi: 10.1161/circulationaha.116.024446.

64 Kirsten A. Herrick, "Iodine Status."

make thyroid hormones. This is one reason for goiter or swelling of the thyroid gland in seriously iodine-deficient individuals.

Now let's take a look at some common symptoms associated with iodine deficiency; some of these are also seen in hypothyroidism (underactive thyroid) because a lack of iodine can slow thyroid gland function and reduce circulating thyroid hormones. And as we discussed, hypothyroidism may be a possible sign of iodine deficiency. But not all causes of hypothyroidism are due to iodine.

Keep in mind the following are just some possible symptoms of iodine deficiency or a thyroid-related disorder. This is not a complete list of all the possible symptoms associated with iodine deficiency or thyroid conditions.

If you're experiencing changes in your health, make an appointment to discuss your symptoms with your doctor, who can provide more information about possible causes for your condition.

Some symptoms include the following:

- sudden weight gain
- tiredness, weakness
- goiter (swelling of the front of the neck)
- hair loss
- feeling cold
- dry skin
- problems with heart rate
- problems with memory and learning
- for women, irregular or heavy menstrual cycles (periods)
- pregnancy-related complications

Since your body may not make enough thyroid hormones when it's low on iodine, this can lead to a slow metabolism and lack of energy because thyroid hormones control many aspects of normal body function like metabolism, growth, development, and the repair of damaged cells.

When your metabolism slows down, you may gain weight because the food you eat is not being converted to energy. This can also lead to tiredness and weakness.

Thyroid hormones also help regenerate hair follicles, and lack of these hormones can cause hair loss. Research has found this happens in those with both a family history of hair loss and those who have an underactive thyroid.

In addition, more than 80 percent of those with an underactive thyroid gland are sensitive to cold temperatures. One reason may be due to a slow metabolism caused by low levels of thyroid hormones.

Iodine deficiency can also cause your heart to beat slower than normal, which if it's severe, can cause dizziness, tiredness, weakness, and even fainting.

Thyroid hormones help your brain grow and develop, especially in early life. However, your body continues to need thyroid hormones throughout various stages of your life for normal function. The part of the brain that controls learning (hippocampus) may be smaller in babies with low thyroid hormone levels.[65]

Severely low thyroid hormone levels (hypothyroidism) can cause a medical emergency called myxedema. This may be life-threatening and requires immediate medical management.

Diagnosis

Symptoms of iodine deficiency can take time to develop. Often people don't know they have an iodine deficiency until they notice neck swelling (goiter) due to thyroid hormone level changes, or it's discovered during a routine medical checkup.

It's important to talk with your doctor if you suspect iodine deficiency or hypothyroidism. Your doctor will likely do blood tests to check

---

65 Gillian E. Cooke, "Hippocampal Volume Is Decreased in Adults with Hypothyroidism," *Thyroid* 24, no. 3 (2014): 433–40, doi: 10.1089/thy.2013.0058.

your thyroid function if you're experiencing certain symptoms of thyroid disease such as sudden weight change, temperature sensitivity, menstrual period–related changes, or goiter. They'll also ask you about your diet to estimate your iodine intake if they suspect you may be deficient.

There are several different tests to check iodine levels and thyroid function, but there are challenges and limitations with each different type of test.[66] Depending on the test, it may be expensive, require inconvenient multiple urine samples, or be inaccurate which can impact treatment decisions. Blood tests, imaging tests, and urine iodine tests done together, along with taking a diet survey of iodine intake, can provide your doctor with a more complete picture of your thyroid health and iodine status.

Urine iodine testing alone can have large variations based on daily iodine intake changes through diet, water, iodized salt use, and other dietary sources.[67] This is why assessing how much iodine you're getting through dietary sources is an important but often overlooked component of checking iodine levels and tailoring diet plans based on iodine intake for better iodine balance, especially for mild to moderate deficiency.

Some options available include the following:

○✕ blood tests to check thyroid function (reliable method)

○✕ 24-hour urine iodine concentration test

○✕ spot urine iodine test

○✕ iodine loading test (not recommended)

○✕ iodine skin patch test (not reliable)

---

66 Patrick Wainwright and Paul Cook, "The Assessment of Iodine Status–Populations, Individuals and Limitations," *Annals of Clinical Biochemistry: International Journal of Laboratory Medicine* 56, no. 1 (2019): 7–14, doi: 10.1177/0004563218774816; Michael B. Zimmermann, "Methods to Assess Iron and Iodine Status," *British Journal of Nutrition* 3 (2008): S2–9, doi: 10.1017/S000711450800679X.

67 Fabian Rohner et al., "Biomarkers of Nutrition for Development–Iodine Review," *The Journal of Nutrition* 144, no. 8 (2014): 1322S–42S, doi: 10.3945/jn.113.181974.

⚮ imaging tests (ultrasound or thyroid scan)

Keep in mind that iodine deficiency is difficult to diagnose, and many types of testing do not provide an accurate reading of your iodine levels. Studies have found urine testing methods used alone are inaccurate in estimating iodine levels.[68] Checking dietary iodine content is an important component that should be included with urine iodine testing to better understand overall iodine levels.

If you have symptoms of iodine deficiency, check with your doctor on testing options. They will assess your complete health to diagnose the cause of your specific symptoms and to guide your treatment, including prescribing medications for a thyroid disorder or iodine supplements if necessary.

Some available tests are not accurate, and relying on those to make decisions about your diet or supplement needs may worsen thyroid-related problems.

Urine Iodine Concentration (UIC) Tests

There are a few types of UIC tests.[69] The spot urine iodine elimination (UIE) test is inexpensive and commonly used for large population-level iodine testing. It provides a quick snapshot of iodine levels. This is often done by public health agencies to determine iodine levels of the general population. However, it is not accurate for measuring individual iodine levels because they can vary a lot.

To get a more accurate picture of urine iodine levels, particularly for individuals, 24-hour urine collection and analysis can provide more comprehensive iodine level data. However, this is more burdensome and expensive. Flaws with this test can occur if the sample is not collected and stored properly before analysis.

---

68 Juan WenYen, "Comparison of 2 Methods for Estimating the Prevalences of Inadequate and Excessive Iodine Intakes," *The American Journal of Clinical Nutrition* 104, no. 3 (2016): 888S–97S, doi: 10.3945/ajcn.115.110346.

69 World Health Organiziation, "Urinary Iodine Concentrations for Determining Iodine Status Deficiency."

Urine iodine levels can change based on the time of collection, fasting state, how much iodine you take in before urine testing, water consumption, and other independent factors.[70] Studies have shown that pre-testing factors can alter UIC levels, meaningfully, posing challenges for health assessments.

For example, one study of children aged 6 through 12 years found those who skipped breakfast before their morning UIC testing had iodine levels that were 40–50 mcg/L lower than those who ate breakfast.[71] A greater number of those children also had levels below 100 mcg/L. Understanding pre-testing factors and accounting for them may improve testing guidelines and interpretation of results.

Urine iodine concentration tests provide an estimate of daily iodine intake. To calculate the daily intake, the following formula is used:

Urinary iodine (micrograms per liter) × 0.0235 × weight (kg) = daily iodine intake.[72] This assumes that 92 percent of iodine is removed from urine in 24 hours.

Example: If a woman weighing 70 kg (about 154 lbs.) has a urine iodine elimination level of 130 mcg/L, her daily iodine intake estimate would be 130 mcg/L x 0.0235 x 70 kg = 214 mcg.

This meets the adult iodine RDA (150 mcg) and is below the maximum limit of 1,100 mcg.

70 Offie Porat Soldin, "Controversies in Urinary Iodine Determinations," *Clinical Biochemistry* 35, no. 8 (2002): 575–9, doi: 10.1016/s0009-9120(02)00406-x; Cria G. Perrine et al., "Comparison of Population Iodine Estimates from 24-Hour Urine and Timed-Spot Urine Samples," *Thyroid* 24, no. 4 (2014): 748–57, doi: 10.1089/thy.2013.0404.

71 Radhouene Doggui, Myriam El Ati-Hellal, Pierre Traissac, and Jalila El Ati, "Pre-Aanalytical Factors Influence Accuracy of Urine Spot Iodine Assessment in Epidemiological Surveys," *Biological Trace Element Research* 186, no. 2 (December 2018): 337–45, doi: 10.1007/s12011-018-1317-y. Epub 2018 Mar 26. PMID: 29582222.

72 Institute of Medicine (US) Panel on Micronutrients, *Dietary Reference Intakes for Vitamin A, Vitamin K, Arsenic, Boron, Chromium, Copper, Iodine, Iron, Manganese, Molybdenum, Nickel, Silicon, Vanadium, and Zinc* (Washington, DC: National Academies Press, 2001), https://www.ncbi.nlm.nih.gov/books/NBK222323.

Your doctor can go over the different types of urine iodine testing and their accuracy. They can also explain why a certain test may be needed and what you can expect with testing.

Iodine-Loading Test

This test requires ingesting a large dose of iodine (50 milligrams) and then collecting all urine for a 24-hour period to test iodine levels. If urine collection is not done correctly or if it's stored improperly, the test is invalid. It is difficult and inconvenient since it requires a full day of urine collection.

It is not an accurate way to measure iodine levels since absorption rates can vary from person to person, and other factors can change the urine iodine concentration.

Iodine Skin Patch Test

The iodine skin patch test is an old test and not accurate to determine iodine levels, although it continues to be popular because it is simple and inexpensive. The false rationale behind this test is based on how quickly iodine solution placed on the skin is absorbed. The theory is this: The faster a patch of iodine solution disappears when applied to the skin, the more deficient you are. And, if it takes 24 hours to disappear, your iodine levels are fine.

This is not scientifically accurate because iodine oxidizes when it's exposed to air and will evaporate as a result. In addition, absorption onto skin varies from person to person and is not an accurate measure of iodine levels. Some iodine is absorbed into skin, but it's impossible to tell your iodine levels or iodine needs based on the skin patch test.

Awareness of Iodine's Role for Your Health

Several public health organizations, including the Endocrine Society, the American Thyroid Association, and the American Academy of Pediatrics, have issued recommendations for pregnant and breast-feeding women to take a multivitamin or mineral supplement that has 150 µg of iodine on a daily basis.[73]

A 2017 survey of 199 midwives and 277 obstetricians in the US found that while one-third believe women to be iodine deficient, a majority of them don't recommend iodine-containing vitamins to those planning pregnancy, during pregnancy, or while breastfeeding.[74] It may also surprise you to learn that only around 60 percent of prenatal vitamins sold in the US contain iodine. The recommendations from the public health organizations haven't been universally adopted.

To be clear, as long as you're eating a balanced diet containing adequate amounts of iodine, this isn't a concern. Population surveys in the US over the past 50 years show that certain groups of people are vulnerable to iodine deficiency and its harmful impact on health. Remember, according to WHO, iodine deficiency is the most common preventable cause of fetal and infant brain developmental disabilities.

---

73 Leslie De Groot, "Management of Thyroid Dysfunction During Pregnancy and Postpartum: An Endocrine Society Clinical Practice Guideline," *The Journal of Clinical Endocrinology and Metabolism* 97, no. 8 (2012): 2543–65, doi: 10.1210/jc.2011-2803; Erik K. Alexander et al., "2017 Guidelines of the American Thyroid Association for the Diagnosis and Management of Thyroid Disease During Pregnancy and the Postpartum," *Thyroid* 27, no. 3 (2017): 315–89, doi: 10.1089/thy.2016.0457; Walter J. Rogan et al., "Iodine Deficiency, Pollutant Chemicals, and the Thyroid: New Information on an Old Problem," *Pediatrics* 133, no. 6 (2014): 1163–66, doi: 10.1542/peds.2014-0900.

74 Simone De Leo et al., "Iodine Supplementation in Women During Preconception, Pregnancy, and Lactation: Current Clinical Practice by U.S. Obstetricians and Midwives," *Thyroid* 27, no. 3 (2017): 434–39, doi: 10.1089/thy.2016.0227.

The CDC nutrition survey (NHANES) finds only around 20 percent of pregnant women and around 15 percent of lactating women in the US take an iodine-containing supplement. Since data show nearly 40 percent of pregnancies are unplanned, it's important for women to understand the crucial role iodine plays in early fetal development and correct deficiencies prior to pregnancy.

The amount of iodine in breast milk can vary based on a mother's diet a few hours before she breastfeeds her baby. Breastfed infants rely on human milk as their sole source of iodine. This can place infants at risk for iodine deficiency and impact their growth and development if a mother's diet is regularly deficient. While a mother's diet impacts the nutrients found in her breast milk—and her baby's nutrition—it's still not clear how much diet is a factor.

When iodine deficiency is suspected in a breastfeeding mother, breast milk is measured for iodine content. And urine iodine levels are measured to learn an infant's or toddler's iodine levels. Urine iodine concentration levels are the simplest test to determine iodine levels but it is not always an accurate measure due to the nature of testing (snapshot). It should not be used exclusively when determining thyroid health or iodine supplementation.

It's challenging to assess iodine levels accurately. The urine iodine test is really just a snapshot of the previous few days. However, currently urine iodine level tests are the easiest procedure to get a general idea of your iodine levels. If your levels are too low or too high, your doctor will likely do other tests to check your thyroid function.

Although international health groups and medical experts have raised concerns that iodine deficiency in mothers who are breastfeeding can affect them and their babies, currently there isn't global consensus on prevention strategies or iodine balancing goals. Women's awareness about the risks of iodine deficiency's impact during pregnancy and while breastfeeding is also low, contributing to that risk.

Given the lifelong consequences of chronically low iodine levels, it is important to understand individual risks, increase your awareness of iodine deficiency causes, and take steps to correct any deficiencies. One step in this process is to learn about your specific risk based on your age, diet, and family history of thyroid disorders. Experts agree that having balanced, normal iodine levels is an important way to prevent thyroid problems.

Awareness of iodine's connection to your overall health can help you manage your diet to maintain adequate levels throughout your life. And if you're planning to become pregnant, or are pregnant, talk with your doctor to make sure you're getting enough iodine and ask them if you need any adjustments to your diet or need to take a multivitamin supplement. If you're concerned about your iodine level, you can ask your doctor to check your level.

CHAPTER 4

Risks of Excess Iodine in the Body

Key Points

⋈ Certain autoimmune thyroid conditions such as Graves' disease or Hashimoto's thyroiditis can make you more sensitive to iodine level changes, triggering an over- or underactive thyroid gland.

⋈ Some types of seaweed such as kelp have the highest natural sources of iodine.

⋈ Iodine poisoning is a rare but serious medical condition that requires immediate medical management.

Most people can tolerate shifts in iodine levels without serious negative health effects, as long as those shifts are temporary. However, if you have a preexisting thyroid condition or have experienced iodine deficiency in the past, you may be more vulnerable to thyroid disorders, such as hyperthyroidism, hypothyroidism, or autoimmune thyroid conditions such as Graves' disease, if you take too much iodine. This may happen even with small increases in iodine intake, but it's particularly risky if you're exposed to high levels of iodine for a long time or experience an iodine overdose.

Pregnant women are also more sensitive to big shifts in iodine levels. Levels above 500 mcg/L are considered excess iodine. A 2021 study (2018–2020) of 515 pregnant women conducted in a city in Hubei Province, China—an area with historical iodine deficiency—

found those with levels above 500 mcg/L had higher amounts of thyroid-stimulating hormone (TSH) and low free T4 levels and were at risk for thyroid disorder.[75]

The study found that women who consumed more iodine-rich foods (seafood, milk, iodized salt) and who took an iodine-containing multivitamin had higher urine iodine levels and higher incidences of thyroid disorder compared with those with low or even more than adequate iodine levels. The study also found that in women with excess iodine levels, early symptoms of mild hypothyroidism were the most common type of thyroid disorder.

Generally, thyroid-related effects from too much iodine are mild and temporary in healthy individuals. But hyperthyroidism from excess iodine can be life-threatening in some people who are sensitive to its effects. It's also important to note that both iodine deficiency and iodine excess can manifest with similar symptoms, making it difficult to discern the actual cause of thyroid-related malfunction. This is why, if you're having symptoms of thyroid problems, you need to check with your doctor and get an accurate diagnosis for your condition. Iodine balance is the key to a properly working thyroid gland. Too much iodine or too little can damage the thyroid gland if it continues long term.

Excess iodine exposure may come from taking iodine supplements such as potassium iodide, taking kelp supplements, eating too many foods with high iodine content (dairy, seafood, etc.), consuming too much iodized salt, being exposed to iodinated radiology contrast dye from medical procedures, or taking a medication called amiodarone for heart-rhythm-related problems.

Amiodarone contains 75 milligrams (mg) of iodine in each 200-mg tablet. It can cause hypothyroidism or thyrotoxicosis (too much thyroid hormone) in some people. Other sources of iodine you may

75 Yuhan Zhou et al., "Establishment of an Iodine Model for Prevention of Iodine-Excess-Induced Thyroid Dysfunction in Pregnant Women," *Open Life Sciences* 16, no. 1 (2021): 1357–64, doi: 10.1515/biol-2021-0142.

not be familiar with include certain cough syrups, prescription medications, mouthwashes, vaginal douches, cosmetics, and nutrition products.

It's not always easy to tell how much iodine we're getting through our diet. Experts suggest that iodine levels greater than 300 mcg (micrograms) are considered excess in children and adults, and greater than 500 mcg is considered excess in pregnant women.[76]

Many foods such as dairy and bread contain iodine that's not listed in the nutrition facts label. Many companies add dough conditioners containing iodine to bread. And milk may also have undisclosed iodine from animal feed sources and iodine-containing disinfectants used during milk processing.[77]

The Food and Drug Administration doesn't regulate iodine use in food products and doesn't require its listing. We'll discuss iodine content of certain foods such as dairy and bread in chapter 7. For now, it's important to know that for most people these sources of iodine are not a cause for concern. But getting too much iodine from food sources may contribute to thyroid problems in the long term if you're susceptible to thyroid conditions already.

Keep in mind that any of the preceding factors may be responsible for raised iodine levels, but it's more likely to happen from a combination of these factors—for example, if you consume a diet high in seafood and take iodine supplements. Also, if your thyroid gland is removed (thyroidectomy) because of tumors, hyperthyroidism, or goiter, your body can become sensitive to excess iodine.

Most types of natural foods aren't high enough in iodine content to cause problems. Typically, people get their daily iodine needs from consuming iodized salt. However, some types of foods, particularly

76 Angela M. Leung and Lewis E. Braverman, "Consequences of Excess Iodine," *Nature Reviews Endocrinology* 10, no. 3 (2014): 136–42, doi: 10.1038/nrendo.2013.251.

77 Kyung Won Lee et al., "Food Group Intakes as Determinants of Iodine Status among US Adult Population," *Nutrients* 8, no. 6 (2016): 325, doi: 10.3390/nu8060325.

seaweed, are high in iodine. Ingesting too much of these foods regularly may worsen existing thyroid issues.

According to the National Institutes of Health Office of Dietary Supplements,[78] there are safe upper limits for iodine intake based on your age. Taking more than these amounts, especially long term, can increase your risk of developing thyroid-related problems and iodine poisoning.

Suggested Maximum Daily Iodine Levels

Age	Daily Iodine Upper Limit
1–3 years	200 mcg
4–8 years	300 mcg
9–13 years	600 mcg
14–18 years	900 mcg
Adults	1,100 mcg

Iodine Fact Sheet, National Institutes of Health, Office of Dietary Supplements

Always talk with your doctor if you have specific questions about your iodine levels and the amount of iodine you're getting from your diet before taking iodine supplements.

In some people who may be susceptible to the effects of excess iodine, iodine supplements can cause goiter, hyperthyroidism, or hypothyroidism. Generally, taking too much iodine in one dose won't cause iodine poisoning, but your risk increases if you continue taking too much iodine, especially if you have an autoimmune thyroid condition.

If you or someone you know has ingested too much iodine, get medical help right away. Iodine poisoning is a serious condition that can be life-threatening.

78 National Institutes of Health, "Iodine," accessed September 7, 2022, https://ods.od .nih.gov/factsheets/iodine-consumer.

Misconceptions About Iodine Needs

There are plenty of books, blogs, and expert commentary advocating for increased daily iodine intake to cure a host of issues including mental fog, depression, anxiety, diabetes, heart irregularities, fatigue, cancer, and more. There are fewer books and writings on the health effects of excess iodine. However, they also exist and advocate for being hyperaware of iodine content in dietary sources as a way to prevent thyroid-related problems.

The truth is, scientists, doctors, and other health experts have different opinions on acceptable iodine intake and the risks and consequences of taking high doses. Globally, there are many different suggestions on ideal iodine consumption and iodine levels to avoid thyroid malfunction.

Experts just don't agree on the amount of iodine we need regularly, adding to confusion and misconceptions on supplementing with iodine. This is unfortunate since both low and high levels of iodine can cause thyroid and other health problems.

This is why, if you're exploring iodine's role in your health, you need to first have an open discussion with your doctor about your health concerns. Don't take iodine supplements without understanding the implications of your thyroid history. For example, do you have a family history of thyroid disease or have an autoimmune thyroid disorder? Taking iodine without checking with your doctor could worsen your thyroid function.

Certainly, science has proven iodine is crucial for normal body function since our cells need iodine to work. And there is some clinical research that has shown iodine also has protective effects against some types of cancer and fibrocystic breast disease (noncancerous lumps in breast tissues). Scientists are also exploring iodine's possible protective role in heart disease and cholesterol levels. And we know iodine is crucial for fetal and early childhood development.

However, just as we've learned that low iodine levels can cause health problems, too much iodine can also cause serious health problems with long-term exposure, particularly if you already have a thyroid condition or serious kidney disease. Iodine poisoning can damage the thyroid gland and cause it to break down. In most cases, if it's a temporary iodine excess, the effects will subside once the levels are corrected. But if you have a thyroid condition, your thyroid gland is extra-sensitive, and you may continue to experience problems, even permanently.

Some research has found those with high iodine levels have higher rates of gastric cancer, and individuals receiving treatment with radioactive iodine for thyroid cancer had higher rates of breast and stomach cancers.[79] However, there are conflicting reports from various studies, making it difficult for scientists to know for certain whether high iodine levels increase the risk for certain types of cancers. More research is needed to understand the long-term effects of excess iodine levels on the body.

If you're experiencing symptoms of thyroid-related problems and feel iodine may be a factor, it's best to make an appointment to get your iodine levels checked before taking iodine supplements on your own. Food and supplement sources of iodine are unreliable because amounts can vary greatly. They may also be contaminated with heavy metals such as arsenic, depending on the source.

One of the challenges with iodine is that it's difficult to gauge how much you're getting daily from dietary sources. But it's possible to estimate whether you're getting adequate amounts based on your

---

79 Mine Gulaboglu, "Blood and Urine Iodine Levels in Patients with Gastric Cancer," *Biological Trace Element Research* 113 (2006): 261–71, doi: 10.1385/BTER:113:3:261; Christopher Kim, "The Risk of Second Cancers After Diagnosis of Primary Thyroid Cancer Is Elevated in Thyroid Microcarcinomas," *Thyroid* 23 (2013): 575–82, doi: 10 .1089/thy.2011.0406.

daily nutrition intake. We'll get into more details on dietary sources of iodine in chapter 7 of the book.

Risk Factors for Developing Iodine Excess

Some people are more susceptible to the effects of too much iodine in their body.

They include the following:

- those with preexisting thyroid conditions
- the elderly
- fetuses (unborn babies)
- newborns
- people with other serious health conditions (kidney disease, diabetes)
- people taking certain medications that increase iodine levels (cough syrups, amiodarone, lithium)
- those with long-standing iodine deficiency
- people ingesting too much iodine from water or food sources

Let's take a look at some thyroid conditions that can be affected by excess iodine.

Graves' Disease

Graves' disease is an autoimmune disorder that causes an overactive thyroid gland (hyperthyroidism). When you have this condition, your immune system makes antibodies called thyroid-stimulating immunoglobulins, which attack healthy thyroid cells. This triggers your thyroid gland to make too much thyroid hormone. Graves' disease is one of the most common causes of hyperthyroidism.

Symptoms of Graves' disease are similar to symptoms of hyperthyroidism.

They include the following:

- goiter
- hand tremors
- sensitivity to heat
- muscle weakness
- nervousness
- fast heart rate (tachycardia)
- trouble sleeping
- weight loss
- irregular periods
- problems becoming pregnant
- Graves' dermopathy (thick, red skin around shins, tops of feet)
- Graves' eye problems (dry eyes, irritation, blurred vision, pain or pressure, light sensitivity)

Your risk for developing Graves' disease is higher if you have another autoimmune condition such as rheumatoid arthritis, type 1 diabetes, Crohn's disease, or another autoimmune disorder.

Hyperthyroidism

Hyperthyroidism has many causes. When it is caused by excess iodine exposure, it is also referred to as Jod-Basedow phenomenon. The condition was discovered in the 1800s in people with endemic goiter. When they were given iodine supplementation, they developed thyroid malfunction (thyrotoxicosis) more commonly than those who didn't have endemic goiter.

The condition may be temporary or long-lasting, and those with Graves' disease, a history of iodine deficiency, or nodular goiter are at higher risk. Toxic nodular goiter can also cause hyperthyroidism.

Symptoms of hyperthyroidism include the following:

- muscle weakness
- anxiety
- insomnia
- depression

⚮ irritability   ⚮ fast heart rate

⚮ sudden weight loss   ⚮ tiredness or fatigue

If you have symptoms of hyperthyroidism, it's important to get medical help right away. A life-threatening condition known as a thyroid storm can happen with uncontrolled hyperthyroidism. As mentioned in chapter 3, this can cause dangerously high blood pressure, heart rate, and body temperature, and even loss of consciousness, which can be fatal if not medically managed promptly.

Hashimoto's Thyroiditis

Hashimoto's thyroiditis is an autoimmune condition that causes hypothyroidism. In the US, it's the most common cause for hypothyroidism, especially in women. With Hashimoto's thyroiditis, the immune system (antibodies and white blood cells) attacks thyroid cells and damages them.

Scientists don't know the exact cause of Hashimoto's thyroiditis but believe genetics may play a role. For example, if you have a family history of autoimmune conditions, such as Graves' disease, Addison's disease (a disease affecting the adrenal glands), type 1 diabetes, rheumatoid arthritis, or others, you may be at increased risk of developing the condition.

If you have Hashimoto's thyroiditis, you shouldn't take iodine supplements or eat too many iodine-containing foods without consulting your doctor or an endocrinologist. It could cause your condition to worsen. It's important to check your iodine levels and discuss the risks and benefits of iodine for you.

Symptoms of Hashimoto's thyroiditis include the following:

⚮ cold sensitivity   ⚮ anxiety

⚮ constipation   ⚮ dry skin

⚮ depression   ⚮ feeling tired, sluggish

- brittle nails
- joint pain
- high cholesterol
- hoarse voice
- heavy or irregular periods
- lower-body muscle weakness
- fertility problems
- hair loss
- weight gain

The condition may develop slowly over time and may not be noticeable at first. Some people may develop a goiter, which is an indication of a thyroid disorder.

If you have Hashimoto's thyroiditis, you may be more sensitive to the effects of too much iodine. People with Hashimoto's thyroiditis may have existing hypothyroidism or eventually develop it.

If your doctor suspects you have Hashimoto's thyroiditis, they'll do blood tests to check for certain antibodies, anti-thyroid peroxidase (anti-TPO), and anti-thyroglobulin (anti-Tg). They may also do ultrasound tests to look for thyroid damage.

Sometimes too much iodine causes your thyroid gland to make extra thyroid hormones. This triggers Wolff-Chaikoff effect, a phenomenon explained by Dr. Jan Wolff and Dr. Israel Lyon Chaikoff in 1948 in the United States. They observed that when rats were given high amounts of iodide, the thyroid gland lowered the amount of thyroid hormones it made as a response. This is a protective effect by the thyroid gland to temporarily halt the gland from making excess thyroid hormones when exposed to high amounts of iodine.

For most people with a normal thyroid gland, this effect of slowed thyroid hormone production is temporary and reverses after 48 hours when iodine levels have normalized. The extra iodine is absorbed by the kidneys and removed through urine. But for people who may already have thyroid gland problems, the effects may last longer or become permanent. Examples include Hashimoto's thyroiditis, Graves' disease, cystic fibrosis, diabetes, and those who have serious kidney problems. Unborn babies are very sensitive to iodine levels during their development, since the endocrine system is forming at this time, and they are more sensitive to high iodine levels from maternal intake.

Failing to adapt to high levels of iodine can lead to hypothyroidism if this failure isn't corrected. Scientists aren't sure why some people can't recover from Wolff-Chaikoff effect, but one theory is that there may be existing thyroid damage that prevents the gland from recovering.

Signs and Symptoms of Iodine Excess

Symptoms of excess iodine can depend on how much iodine was ingested, over what time period, if there are preexisting thyroid-related conditions, and your overall health condition.

Too much iodine can cause your pituitary gland to make excessive amounts of thyroid-stimulating hormone (TSH), because it senses low levels of thyroid hormones. This can lead to hyperthyroidism or hypothyroidism and other serious long-term problems.

Keep in mind that these are some possible symptoms of iodine excess. You may experience symptoms different from those listed here. If you're experiencing health-related problems, it's always a good idea to check with your doctor about your symptoms. They can get a complete health history to provide an accurate diagnosis based on your particular symptoms.

Mild symptoms may include the following:

- diarrhea
- nausea
- vomiting
- rash
- fever
- headache
- abdominal pain
- burning sensation in the mouth
- metallic taste in the mouth
- reproductive problems

Serious symptoms may include the following:

- ✕ weak pulse
- ✕ hyperthyroidism
- ✕ throat swelling
- ✕ serious bleeding
- ✕ turning blue (cyanosis)
- ✕ coma

If you have a preexisting heart condition, hyperthyroidism may worsen this condition.

Thyroid Cancer

Thyroid cancer is the most common form of cancer affecting the endocrine system. It accounts for around 2 percent of all new cancers diagnosed in the US, estimated to be about 43,800 new cases annually. Although it is a rare type of cancer, thyroid cancer is reportedly the fifth most common form of cancer in women in the United States.[80] Risk factors for thyroid cancer include exposure to radiation from nuclear fallout, family history of thyroid disorders, radiation therapy in infancy or early childhood, history of goiter, having certain genetic mutations, and being of Asian heritage.

Iodine's role in thyroid cancer is controversial. There is still much we don't know about the connection between high iodine levels and the risk for thyroid cancer. Is it protective or harmful? But what we do know is that iodine balance is important for normal thyroid function. Too much or too little iodine can trigger problems with thyroid hormone levels. Goiter can be caused by either iodine deficiency or iodine excess.

There have been some studies that show excess iodine can cause thyroid cancer, especially papillary thyroid cancer.[81] While there are several different types of thyroid cancer, papillary thyroid cancer is

80 Kenny Lee et al., "Thyroid Cancer," in *StatPearls* (Treasure Island, FL: StatPearls Publishing, 2022).

81 Michikawa Takehiro et al., "Seaweed Consumption and the Risk of Thyroid Cancer in Women the Japan Public Health Center-Based Prospective Study," *European Journal Cancer Prevention* 21, no. 3 (2012): 254–60, doi: 10.1097/CEJ.0b013e32834a8042.

the most common form. It accounts for around 80 percent of thyroid cancers in the United States. It typically grows slowly and affects the follicular cells of the thyroid.

Research in Denmark and China has shown an increased risk of developing thyroid cancer from taking iodine supplements. However, other studies have contradicted this and shown iodine to have a protective role in preventing thyroid cancer, with no association between high seaweed (rich iodine content) intake and thyroid cancer risk.[82] So it's unclear what role iodine levels play in thyroid cancer.

A review of studies found taking 300 mcg or more of iodine and consuming a diet high in saltwater fish and shellfish had a protective effect on thyroid cancer risk.[83] But the results were not clear-cut. In the review, only three of the included studies measured the exact amount of iodine people consumed; other studies relied on calculations based on the average iodine content in specific foods. So, it's difficult to say what factors led to the protective effects. More research is needed to understand if there's a link between excess iodine and thyroid cancer, or if iodine has a protective effect.

Dietary Influences

As we mentioned previously, most types of natural foods don't have high levels of iodine, but some types of food do have higher amounts. For example, seaweed contains some of the highest amounts of iodine.

---

82 Ling-Zhi Cao, "The Relationship Between Iodine Intake and the Risk of Thyroid Cancer: A Meta-Analysis," *Medicine (Baltimore)* 96, no. 20 (2017): E6734, doi: 10.1097 /MD.0000000000006734; Chaochen Wang et al., "Prospective Study of Seaweed Consumption and Thyroid Cancer Incidence in Women: The Japan Collaborative Cohort Study," *European Journal of Cancer Prevention* 25, no. 3 (2016): 239–45, doi: 10.1097 /CEJ.0000000000000168.

83 Ling-Zhi Cao, "The Relationship Between Iodine Intake and the Risk of Thyroid Cancer."

There are wide ranges in iodine content between different seaweed products. The iodine amount depends on the type of seaweed (brown, green, red) and where it grows. Different types of seaweed grow in oceans, lakes, rivers, and other water bodies all over the world. Seaweed is also cultivated in farms in many countries.

On average, seaweed may have iodine ranging from 16 mcg per gram to 2,984 mcg per gram or more, based on the dry weight of seaweed. The table below lists some common locations where seaweed is cultivated. It's not an exhaustive list of all sources of different types of seaweed.

Types of Seaweed and Approximate Iodine Content

Seaweed Name	Type	Cultivated	Iodine Content
Arame *Eisenia bicyclis*	Brown algae	Japan, South Korea	586 mcg per gram
Dulse *Palmaria palmata*	Red algae	Northern Ireland, Canada	72 mcg per gram
Hijiki *Hizikia fusiforme*	Brown algae	Japan, China, South Korea, coastal areas of Northwest Pacific Ocean	629 mcg per gram
Kombu *Laminaria sp.*	Brown algae	Japan	1,350 mcg per gram
Nori *Porphyra tenera*	Red algae	Japan, China, South Korea	16 mcg per gram
Wakame *Alaria esculenta*	Brown algae	Japan, South Korea, Australia	110 mcg to 431 mcg per gram

The table lists general ranges of iodine content based on country of origin, although it's difficult to know exact amounts since processing and seasonal factors can change levels dramatically.

Food sources of iodine can vary significantly from batch to batch, based on country of origin and other influences.[84]

Different varieties of seaweed have been an essential part of the diet of Japan and other Asian countries for thousands of years. As seaweed gains popularity in Western populations, some varieties are grown or cultivated for commercial use in Canada, Europe, and the United States. Seaweed is also grown and farmed in several other countries, including Phillipines, Indonesia, Australia, and others.

For many years, scientists around the world have been studying the many healthful effects of types of seaweed due to its antioxidant, anti-inflammatory, anticancer, antibacterial, and immune defense properties. The varieties kombu and arame have the highest levels of antioxidants, based on research. Antioxidant concentrations of seaweed can depend on where it's cultivated, when it's harvested, and the processing techniques used.

In laboratory tests, kombu had the strongest antibacterial effects against gram-positive bacteria such as *Enterococcus faecalis*. This is a common species of bacteria that lives harmlessly in your intestines. However, for those who may have health conditions or a compromised immune system, it can spread to other areas of the body, including the blood, and cause serious infections. Other common types of seaweed such as wakame, arame, dulse, and hijiki had moderate to weak anti-infective effects on different types of bacteria, viruses, and fungi.[85]

But there is also concern among health experts about heavy metals such as lead, cadmium, and arsenic found in seaweed

---

84 Jane Teas et al., "Variability of Iodine Content in Common Commercially Available Edible Seaweeds," *Thyroid* 14, no. 10 (2004): 836–41, doi: 10.1089/thy.2004.14.836.

85 Natalia Čmiková, "Determination of Antioxidant, Antimicrobial Activity, Heavy Metals and Elements Content of Seaweed Extracts," *Plants (Basel)* 11, no. 11 (2022): 1493, doi: 10.3390/plants11111493.

and the possible negative health effects with frequent, regular consumption. This continues to draw the interest of scientists.

What research has shown so far is that heavy metal amounts in naturally grown seaweed tend to depend on the season. Concentrations are generally lower in summer months, when they grow faster, than in winter months, when growth is slower, causing a buildup of metals. Aluminum and arsenic are commonly found in most types of seaweed, and amounts can vary depending on species, where it's grown, time of harvest, and processing methods used.

Future research needs to examine the impact of environmental contamination on seaweed and how to grow these nutrient-rich foods more sustainably, free of heavy metal contamination, since their popularity as a culinary ingredient continues to grow globally.

Popular Types of Seaweed

Arame (*Eisenia bicyclis*)—native to Japan but also grown in South Korea. It is categorized as brown algae. It's popular in Japanese cuisine and has a mild, sweet flavor. It is typically sold in dried form. It's available in some health food stores, in natural food stores, and online. It is rich in iodine and a good source of iron, calcium, magnesium, and vitamin A. Arame is also high in lignan (phytoestrogen), which has antioxidant benefits. It is also a good source of protein and fiber.

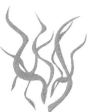

Arame

Dulse (*Palmaria palmata*)—grows naturally in the North Atlantic and Pacific regions. It is native to Northern Ireland. Dulse is categorized as a red algae. It looks like red leaf lettuce when it is fresh. It is typically harvested in the summer months from June to around October. It can

Dulse

be eaten alone or added to various foods such as soups, curries, and even baked goods. Dulse is sold dried, powdered, or in flaked forms in many health food stores and organic groceries. It is also available online for purchase. It is a good source of iodine, calcium, magnesium, iron, B vitamins, vitamin A, and several other minerals. Dulse is also a good source of protein and fiber and is rich in antioxidants.

Hijiki (*Hizikia fusiforme*)—grows naturally in the coastal areas of the northwest Pacific Ocean. It is a type of brown algae that's popular for its nutritional and medicinal properties in China, North and South Korea, Japan, and other Southeast Asian countries. It is also cultivated in South Korea and China.

Hijiki has become popular in the pharmaceutical industry due to the discovery of its many beneficial compounds such as fucoidan, fucosterol, polysaccharides, and phenols.[86] They have anti-tumor, anti-inflammatory, antioxidant, immunomodulatory, and other cell protective properties.

Hijiki

Hijiki has high levels of iodine and also contains other minerals such as calcium, magnesium, potassium, iron, and zinc. It is available in health food stores, in Asian markets, and online.

While hijiki has many potential beneficial properties, it's important to be aware that this seaweed also has higher levels of inorganic arsenic. A 2019 study of Japanese children and pregnant women who consumed hijiki found they had elevated arsenic levels.[87]

86 Maria Dyah Nur Meinita et al., "Hizikia Fusiformis: Pharmacological and Nutritional Properties," *Foods* 10, no. 7 (2021): 1660, doi: 10.3390/foods10071660.

87 Nathan Mise et al., "Hijiki Seaweed Consumption Elevates Levels of Inorganic Arsenic Intake in Japanese Children and Pregnant Women," *Food Additives & Contaminants* 36, no. 1 (2019): 84–95, doi: 10.1080/19440049.2018.1562228.

Kombu (Laminaria sp.)—naturally found in coastal areas of Japan. It is a brown algae variety of kelp that is an elemental part of Japanese and East Asian cuisine. There are several varieties of kombu, and its flavor profile depends on the type. It is available dried and may be eaten on its own or added to soups and other foods to enrich flavor profiles. It is commonly available in health food stores, in Asian markets, and online. It is harvested seasonally in the summer months from June to September.

Kombu

Kombu is high in iodine content. It is a good source of micronutrients such as calcium, magnesium, iron, potassium, zinc, and more. It is also a good source of antioxidants, fiber, and protein. Boiling kombu for 15 to 30 minutes dramatically reduces its iodine levels.

Nori (Porphyra tenera)—the most popular and widely known type of seaweed around the world. It is a type of red algae and is cultivated in Japan, China, and South Korea for commercial sale. It is typically sold dried as sheets and is available in many grocery stores and online. Nori is commonly used to wrap sushi but is also used to add flavor to soups and foods.

Nori

Though nori is not as rich in iodine as other types of seaweeds, it is still considered a good source of iodine as well as other vitamins and minerals including vitamins A, B, and C, zinc, iron, magnesium, calcium, and more.

Like some other types of seaweed, nori may also be contaminated with heavy metals such as arsenic or cadmium.

Wakame (Alaria esculenta)—a type of brown algae that's naturally found around the Australian coast. It is also cultivated for commercial use in Japan and South Korea. It is

Wakame

eaten alone as a snack or used as a seasoning in soups or salads. It's easily available in Asian markets, in organic food stores, and online. It is a good source of fiber and protein, and it contains micronutrients such as iodine, magnesium, iron, and more.

Wakame may also contain arsenic and other heavy metals. The amounts can vary based on where it's grown, where it's harvested, and the processing used for commercial sale.

Thyroid Effects of Seaweed Consumption

Seaweed is a part of the regular diet in Japan, and data indicate around 21 percent of meals contain some type of seaweed.[88] There are at least 20 different species of seaweed popular for regular consumption in Japan containing various amount of iodine. Experts estimate the Japanese people consume the highest amounts of seaweed in the world, an average iodine consumption between 1,000 and 3,000 mcg per day.

Some research indicates high consumption of seaweed among Japanese populations may contribute to their good health and long life. But scientists don't yet know if it's all good or if there may be some downside due to contamination when high amounts are consumed for long periods of time.

Boiling seaweed can drastically reduce its iodine content. For example, boiling kombu for 15 minutes causes it to lose 99 percent of its iodine. It's unclear if the methods and uses of seaweed in Japan provide different effects.

Kombu (kelp) has one of the highest amounts of iodine, and the range can vary widely depending on the country of origin, from

---

88 Theordore T. Zava and David T. Zava, "Assessment of Japanese Iodine Intake Based on Seaweed Consumption in Japan: A Literature-Based Analysis," *Thyroid Research* 4, no. 14 (2011), doi: 10.1186/1756-6614-4-14.

1,300 to 8,000 mcg per gram in kelp flakes. Wakame and nori are more popular and consumed more often than kelp. There have been several reports of serious thyroid problems caused by consuming high doses of kelp in many countries.

While iodine needs increase during pregnancy, there have been several reports of hypothyroidism in babies whose moms took iodine supplements or consumed excessive amounts of seaweed products while they were pregnant. The American Thyroid Association advises against taking daily iodine supplements or products with levels above 500 mcg, except under medical supervision for certain medical conditions.

It's important to discuss your diet and iodine intake with your doctor before eating too much seaweed or other iodine-containing supplements. Certainly, if you have an underlying thyroid condition, taking too much seaweed may affect you differently than if you have normal thyroid function. It's always a good idea to talk with your doctor before drastically changing your diet.

Diagnosis of Excess Iodine

Iodine poisoning is rare, but it may happen in some cases from taking dietary supplements or other products with very high iodine amounts. In most cases, with a normal thyroid gland, excess iodine is eliminated and doesn't pose problems in the long term. However, some people are more vulnerable to risks from too much iodine.

If you or someone you know has taken too much iodine, get medical help immediately. Iodine poisoning is a serious condition that requires medical care.

If you have symptoms of hyperthyroidism or hypothyroidism from excess iodine consumption, your doctor will do certain tests to check your levels. They include the following:

 ✗ blood tests to check thyroid function (a reliable test)

- urine iodine creatinine ratio test
- serum iodine test
- imaging tests to check your thyroid gland such as a thyroid ultrasound or a radioactive iodine uptake test

We've already discussed different types of iodine level tests available for different scenarios. There are also some tests that are more useful and preferred when checking for iodine excess or iodine poisoning. If you have symptoms of iodine excess, talk with your doctor about getting your levels checked.

Urine Iodine Creatinine Ratio Test

The urine iodine creatinine ratio test may be used to evaluate iodine levels when high iodine levels or iodine poisoning is suspected. It can also be useful to determine the success of a low-iodine diet in people on radioactive iodine treatment.[89]

There are limitations to the accuracy of this test in certain circumstances. Creatinine is a muscle-waste product of creatine (protein) that's removed through your kidneys. Creatinine levels can vary based on your metabolism, how much meat you consume, and your age.

In some cases, such as with kidney disease, muscle wasting, older age, or increased water consumption, creatinine levels can change and affect urine iodine creatinine levels. It's also difficult to collect urine creatinine because it can degrade if it's not stored properly before a specimen is analyzed.

89 Hee Kyung Kim et al., "Usefulness of Iodine/Creatinine Ratio from Spot-Urine Samples to Evaluate the Effectiveness of Low-Iodine Diet Preparation for Radioiodine Therapy," *Clinical Endocrinology* 73, no. 1 (2010): 114–8, doi: *10.1111/j.1365-2265.2009 .03774.x.*

To learn more about this type of test and its uses, ask your doctor about its accuracy, its costs, and how it's done.

Serum Iodine Test

Serum iodine testing is a reliable blood test that's frequently used to check for excess iodine. It is often administered along with thyroid blood tests and urine iodine concentration tests.[90] The main components of a serum iodine test are iodide and iodine in thyroxine. The normal suggested ranges are between 64 and 154 nanomoles per liter. This includes around 33 to 79 mcg/L of iodine, which is the biggest part of a serum iodine reading.

Studies have shown serum iodine levels match up with urine iodine concentration tests when someone has excess iodine levels.[91] The intestine absorbs excess iodine to slow its absorption in the body. Some excess is also removed through urine. Another study found higher goiter rates (5 percent) in children 7 to 10 years of age when their iodine intake was greater than 250 mcg/L, and higher goiter rates in children 11 to 14 years when their iodine intake was higher than 300 mcg/L.

If your doctor feels this type of iodine testing is needed, they'll explain the rationale for using the serum iodine test, how it's done, the costs, and what you can expect.

90 Tingkai Cui et al., "Serum Iodine Is Correlated with Iodine Intake and Thyroid Function in School-Age Children from a Sufficient-to-Excessive Iodine Intake Area," *The Journal of Nutrition* 149, no. 6 (2019): 1012–18, doi: 10.1093/jn/nxy325.

91 Xing Jin et al., "The Application of Serum Iodine in Assessing Individual Iodine Status," *Clinical Endocrinology* 87, no. 6 (2017): 807–14, doi: 10.1111/cen.13421; Wen Chen et al., "Associations Between Iodine Intake, Thyroid Volume, and Goiter Rate in School-Aged Chinese Children from Areas with High Iodine Drinking Water Concentrations," *American Journal of Clinical Nutrition* 105, no. 1 (2017): 228–33, doi: 10.3945/ajcn.116.139725.

CHAPTER 5

Benefits of Iodine Balance for Your Health

The truth is that our understanding of iodine's role in health is still evolving, and scientists are learning new information through research every day. While experts may not agree on how much iodine is beneficial for health, they all agree that adequate iodine levels are essential for normal thyroid function.

One of the challenges with iodine is that it's not easy to accurately gauge how much we're getting, based on food or water sources. And it can also take a while for symptoms of deficiency or excess to show up, complicating a diagnosis of iodine imbalance.

Iodine and Your Health

Iodine has a host of benefits and directly or indirectly affects growth, metabolism, and development, beginning in early life and continuing throughout different life stages. Iodine's benefits are principally connected to its effects on the thyroid gland, but research has also found iodine has antioxidant, anti-infective, and potential anticancer effects.[92]

---

92 Salvatore Sorrenti et al., "Iodine: Its Role in Thyroid Hormone Biosynthesis and Beyond," *Nutrients* 3, no. 12 (2021): 4469, doi: 10.3390/nu13124469.

Scientists believe iodine's beneficial effects happen through a variety of biochemical pathways.[93] And it is found in organs other than the thyroid. For example, it's found in the prostate, pancreas, ovaries, and mammary glands. In addition, iodine is also possibly in the immune system, nervous system, and gastric system.

Antioxidant Effects

Oxidative stress refers to an imbalance between antioxidants and free radicals in your body. While your body needs some free radicals for healing wounds and other crucial body functions, too many free radicals can damage cells, causing or worsening various health problems.

Research has shown that too many free radicals can cause age-related chronic (long-standing) degenerative and inflammatory conditions.

They include the following:[94]

- cancer
- heart disease and stroke
- lipid disorders (cholesterol, triglycerides)
- diabetes
- respiratory conditions (asthma)
- joint disease
- kidney disease
- liver disease

93 Carmen Aceves et al., "Molecular Iodine Has Extrathyroidal Effects as an Antioxidant, Differentiator, and Immunomodulator," *International Journal of Molecular Sciences* 22, no. 3 (2021): 1228, doi: 10.3390/ijms22031228; Carmen Aceves, Brenda Anguiano, and Guadalupe Delgado, "The Extrathyronine Actions of Iodine as Antioxidant, Apoptotic, and Differentiation Factor in Various Tissues," *Thyroid* 23, no. 8 (2013): 938–46, doi: 10.1089/thy.2012.0579.

94 Andrew W. Caliri, Stella Tommasi, and Ahmad Besaratinia, "Relationships Among Smoking, Oxidative Stress, Inflammation, Macromolecular Damage, and Cancer," *Reviews in Mutation Research*, no. 787 (2021): 108365, doi: 10.1016/j.mrrev.2021 .108365; Gabriele Pizzino, "Oxidative Stress: Harms and Benefits for Human Health," *Oxidative Medicine and Cellular Longevity*, no. 2017 (2017), doi: 10.1155/2017 /8416763; Sha Li et al., "The Role of Oxidative Stress and Antioxidants in Liver Diseases," *International Journal of Molecular Sciences* 16, no. 11 (2015): 26,087–124, doi: 10.3390/ijms161125942.

- neurological conditions (Alzheimer's disease, dementia)
- eye disease (macular degeneration, glaucoma, dry eyes, cataract)

If you have oxidative stress you may experience the following:

- fatigue
- memory problems
- infections
- faster aging (wrinkles, gray hair)

Antioxidants can bind to free radicals and counteract their damaging effects. Certain environmental and lifestyle factors such as pollution, cigarette smoke, sun exposure, some medications, obesity, radiation, pesticides, or chemicals can increase the number of free radicals in your body. Long term, this causes oxidative stress and tissue and cellular damage.

Research shows iodine has antioxidant and anti-infective properties, and it also binds free radicals. These actions allow iodine to have protective and disease prevention benefits for different areas of the body in addition to the thyroid gland.[95]

Older research studies have shown iodine has antioxidant properties in doses higher than 1 milligram (mg) per day. And studies have also found molecular iodine in concentrations from 1 to 6 mg per day has protective effects against certain benign conditions such as fibrocystic breast disease, ovarian cysts, and prostatic hyperplasia (enlarged prostate gland). Fibrocystic breast disease is a benign (noncancerous) condition affecting millions of women that causes painful lumps to form in breast tissue. Scientists believe hormonal changes and genetics are a factor in the condition.

In studies, people who received iodine treatments (1 mg to 6 mg) from five weeks to up to two years experienced benefits in condi-

---

95 Rudolf Winkler, "Iodine—A Potential Antioxidant and the Role of Iodine/Iodide in Health and Disease," *Natural Science* 7, no. 12 (2015): 548–57, doi: 10.4236/ns.2015 .712055.

tions such as fibrocystic breast disease and prostatic hyperplasia without side effects.

However, patients who received higher doses of iodine (9 mg or 12 mg per day) did experience some side effects including temporary hypothyroidism, headache, diarrhea, acne, and sinus inflammation or infection (sinusitis). These side effects resolved once the high dose of iodine was stopped.

More research is needed to understand iodine's protective effects in the body at different levels before universal supplementation can be supported. If you have signs of oxidative stress, talk with your doctor about your diet, nutrition, and lifestyle. Ask them about checking your thyroid function and your iodine levels.

Note: There is not enough information about the safety of high iodine ingestion during pregnancy or in newborns. This is why experts recommend not exceeding the recommended upper limits of iodine for these groups. If you have questions about how much iodine is safe to take during pregnancy, talk with your doctor or pharmacist. They can guide you on safe limits.

Anticancer Effects

Iodine's potential anticancer effects have been debated by scientists for many years. Data from some research studies show that people whose diet includes iodine-rich foods have lower incidences of certain types of cancers. Conversely, other research has also shown high iodine levels may contribute to thyroid problems and increase some cancer risk. This is confusing! It means we need better-designed studies to learn more about iodine's potential protective effects against some types of cancer.

For example, as we emphasized on page 98, types of seaweed are very high in iodine, and certain Asian cultures consume high amounts as part of their daily diet. Research shows the Japanese culture consumes more than 25 times the amount of seaweed as Western populations, and some studies show the Japanese have lower rates of breast and prostate cancer.

Studies in animals and humans have found iodine supplements curb tumor growth and development—both benign and cancerous. Eastern medical practitioners have been using iodine-rich foods to treat breast cancer and shrink tumors and nodules for many years.

Other research shows iodine causes apoptosis or programmed cell death of various types of cancer cells through direct and indirect actions on cells. One intriguing theory is that cancer cells may be more sensitive to effects of iodine because research has found that types of tumors have higher levels of arachidonic acid (an inflammatory essential fatty acid). Too much arachidonic acid can cause inflammatory responses in the body from prostaglandin release.

Scientists have found cancer cells are more vulnerable to apoptosis from iodine exposure than normal cells. They believe this is one way iodine may have anticancer effects. Other cancer cells that seem susceptible to iodine include lung, pancreas, prostate, skin, nerve, spine, and brain cancer cells.

However, different studies have found conflicting results. Some studies have suggested iodine has protective effects against breast cancer, and that it lowers rates of fibrocystic breast disease.[96] Various international studies have found iodine deficiency increases the risk for breast cancer and breast fibroids. Yet other research has found higher incidences of breast, stomach, and thyroid cancers in individuals with high iodine levels.

The bottom line is that we need more data to confirm the benefits of iodine for various types of cancer. Experts are also exploring what

---

96 Saeed Kargar et al., "Urinary Iodine Concentrations in Cancer Patients," *Asian Pacific Journal of Cancer Prevention* 18, no. 3 (2017): 819–21, doi: 10.22034/APJCP.2017 .18.3.819; Shaohua He, "Iodine Stimulates Estrogen Receptor Singling and Its Systemic Level Is Increased in Surgical Patients Due to Topical Absorption," *Oncotarget* 9, no. 1 (2018): 375–84, doi: 10.18632/oncotarget.2063.

dosages of iodine may offer protective benefits versus causing harmful effects.

This is why it's important not to supplement with iodine on your own. If you have a family history of cancer and you're wondering if taking iodine would be beneficial, talk with your doctor. They can tell you more about the pros and cons of iodine supplements and what the latest research shows.

Anti-infective

Iodine's antiseptic properties have been recognized for hundreds of years. Lugol's solution was the first iodine-based antiseptic used for wound care. It became popular for its antiseptic benefits during the American Civil War and was used until the 1950s, when newer antiseptic formulations were introduced. The early Lugol's solution had some drawbacks. It caused pain and irritation when it was applied to wounds, and it stained the skin, making it less desirable for wound care. However, newer iodine-based solutions such as povidone-iodine are gentler for wound care, and still used today.[97]

Iodine has been shown to be an effective antiseptic against a broad range of pathogens such as bacteria, viruses, molds, yeasts, and protozoa. Iodine has been effective at preventing growth of certain resistant bacteria such as methicillin-resistant staphylococci and biofilm forms of *Pseudomonas aeruginosa*, which are resistant to many available anti-infective treatments.

It has demonstrated superior antiseptic qualities over some traditional wound-care antiseptics such as silver sulfadiazine.[98] However, experts believe iodine may not be suitable for those with

---

97 Rose Cooper, "Iodine Revisited," *International Wound Journal* 4, no. 2 (2007): 124–37, doi: 10.1111/j.1742-481X.2007.00314.x.

98 H. Vermeulen, S. J. Westerbos, and D. T. Ubbink, "Benefit and Harm of Iodine in Wound Care: A Systematic Review, *Journal of Hospital Infection* 76, no. 3 (2010): 191–9, doi: 10.1016/j.jhin.2010.04.026.

thyroid problems, pregnant or lactating women, or newborns. This is because very little safety data exist on iodine use in these groups. Experts also recommend against using iodine products to treat large burn wounds or in those with serious kidney problems.

Today, iodine-derived antiseptic products are mainly used to clean or disinfect skin wounds to lower the risks of surface bacterial growth and infection.

Immune Booster

Food and nutrition have long been recognized as crucial components of good health. Our bodies need vitamins and minerals for normal growth and development. But it's more than that. Lack of nutrients can cause our immune system to falter. It can make us more prone to certain illnesses and susceptible to autoimmune conditions and other chronic health disorders.

Our immune system has two main modes to fight off foreign pathogens. The first is called a *natural immune response*. This response system is an immediate defense alert system that responds when it senses a foreign substance such as a virus, bacteria, or other foreign pathogen is invading the body. The second type of immune response is called an *adaptive immune response*. This is when T and B cells (lymphocytes—white blood cells) recognize antigens in foreign matter and generate antibodies to fight and destroy them. They also recruit other immune defenders to fight the invader.[99]

Your nutritional status is key to fighting certain types of illnesses such as bacterial or viral diarrhea, pneumonia, measles, and more. However, nutrition isn't a factor in your body's vulnerability to other types of infections such as HIV, viral encephalitis, influenza, or tetanus. Basically, studies have shown vitamins and minerals help

99 Saikat Mitra et al., "Exploring the Immune-Boosting Functions of Vitamins and Minerals as Nutritional Food Bioactive Compounds: A Comprehensive Review," *Molecule* 27, no. 2 (2022): 555, doi: 10.3390/molecules27020555.

boost your immune system to resist some infections and immune recovery.

Research has shown iodide has immune-boosting effects and may assist the immune system by expressing anti-tumor effects, increasing the immune system's ability to defend against foreign pathogens, and clearing infections.[100] But more evidence is needed to understand how iodine provides immune-boosting effects on various body systems.

Immunomodulators are natural substances made by your immune system to keep you healthy and defend against invaders. There are several different types of immunomodulators with different immune-related functions. These synthetic or biological compounds either boost, stimulate, or slow parts of the immune system as a response mechanism. There are three types of immunomodulators; they are classified based on how they work. They include immuno-suppressants, immunostimulants, and immunoadjuvants. Immuno-suppressants tamp down the actions of the immune system to calm it for autoimmune disorders, immunostimulants help activate or increase parts of the immune system, and immunoadjuvants boost immune function.

Iodine acts as an immunomodulator through its anti-infective properties. Scientists believe iodine may help the immune system by removing chemicals and toxins from the body and tamping down certain autoimmune reactions in the body. This helps improve how your immune system works. Research has also shown thyroid hormones influence the immune system by activating anti-tumor effects, and iodine levels influence thyroid hormone activities.

100 Mahmood Y. Bilal et al., "A Role for Iodide and Thyroglobulin in Modulating the Function of Human Immune Cells. Front Immunol," *Frontiers in Immunology* 8, no. 1573 (2017), doi: 10.3389/fimmu.2017.01573.

CHAPTER 6

Thyroid Conditions and Treatments

So far, you've read about how your diet, age, and other factors can impact your iodine levels. You're also familiar with symptoms associated with iodine deficiency and excess. But thyroid disorders may also be caused by autoimmune conditions and other influences such as family history, certain medications, treatment for thyroid cancer, or a thyroid disorder—not just iodine.

Treatment options for various thyroid conditions depend on the cause and level of the thyroid disorder. In some cases, your doctor may opt just to monitor your thyroid function and treat you if it becomes necessary.

In this chapter, we'll talk about different types of thyroid conditions and their treatments, including iodine-related changes that affect thyroid gland function.

Remember, if you're experiencing specific symptoms of thyroid disorders, it's best to speak with a trained medical professional. Don't assume iodine is the cause of your thyroid problem. Your doctor will order tests to diagnose the cause, and they'll go over the various treatment options and the effectiveness of each for your condition based on your diagnosis.

Always ask about what you can expect with treatment including side effects, timeline, and the outlook for your condition.

Let's take a look at some types of thyroid conditions, symptoms, diagnoses, and possible treatment options.

Keep in mind that these are not all the possible causes of thyroid-related problems and their treatments. Your doctor will discuss your individual circumstance and what's appropriate for you. This includes diagnosing iodine deficiency and discussing dietary solutions. Here is a look at thyroid conditions.

Hypothyroidism

Your thyroid gland is underactive and doesn't make enough thyroid hormones. This may be caused by iodine deficiency, Hashimoto's thyroiditis (an autoimmune condition), radioiodine treatment for hyperthyroidism, surgery to remove the thyroid gland, pituitary gland or hypothalamus disorders, taking certain medications, thyroiditis, or congenital hypothyroidism.

Symptoms include the following:

- constipation
- depression
- dry skin and hair
- tiredness
- heavy or irregular periods, problems with fertility
- cold sensitivity
- memory problems
- slow heart rate
- weight gain

Diagnosis

The diagnosis for hypothyroidism usually involves blood tests to check thyroid hormone levels and imaging tests to check the thyroid gland. They include checking T4 (thyroxine) and TSH (thyroid-stimulating hormone). If your thyroxine levels are low and your TSH levels are high, you may have hypothyroidism. It could also mean your pituitary gland is making too much TSH to stimulate your thyroid gland to make more thyroid hormones.

If you have symptoms of Hashimoto's thyroiditis, as described in chapters 3 and 4, your doctor will order blood tests to check thyroid hormone levels, T4 levels, and T3 levels. And because Hashimoto's is an autoimmune condition, they'll also check to see if you have an unusual number of antibodies that might be attacking your thyroid gland. There is currently no cure for Hashimoto's thyroiditis.

Treatments

The treatment for hypothyroidism depends on the cause. If hypothyroidism is caused by iodine deficiency, balancing iodine levels can normalize thyroid function. Your doctor will discuss your diet and other sources of iodine to help balance your levels. It's important to keep iodine levels adequate to avoid thyroid problems. Other nutrients such as zinc, selenium, vitamin D, and vitamin B12 have also been linked to hypothyroidism. It's important to have adequate levels of these nutrients as well.

Treatments for other causes of hypothyroidism, including Hashimoto's thyroiditis, involve taking a medication known as *levothyroxine*. It is a synthetic thyroid hormone that helps your body make T4 (thyroxine). In some people, taking it regularly can help the thyroid gland to function normally.

Levothyroxine is also used to suppress TSH levels as part of a thyroid cancer treatment regimen after surgery.

The dosage of levothyroxine depends on the cause of hypothyroidism and the thyroid gland's ability to function. The medication is taken by mouth once per day. Your dosage may be adjusted every four to six weeks initially until your levels are stable. As long as you're on a thyroid hormone, you'll need to have routine blood tests that check your hormone levels to make sure you stay within a good range so you avoid major shifts that can cause hyperthyroidism.

Certain foods, medications, or supplements can interfere with how levothyroxine works and make it less effective or increase the risk of side effects.

This is not a complete list of all possible interactions with levothyroxine. Talk to your doctor or pharmacist for more information if you're prescribed levothryoxine. They can tell you about all the side effects and interactions.

Some interactions with levothyroxine include the following:

- antidepressants (amitriptyline)—may increase the side effects of both medications
- antiseizure medications (carbamazepine, phenytoin)—can reduce the effect of levothyroxine
- blood thinners (warfarin)—increase the risk of bleeding
- calcium supplements—can reduce the effect of levothyroxine
- proton-pump inhibitors for acid reflux like esomeprozole (Nexium), omeprazole (Prilosec), lansoprazole (Prevacid)—can reduce the effect of levothyroxine if taken together
- rifampin (antibiotic)—can reduce the effect of levothyroxine

Another type of thyroid medication known as desiccated (dried) thyroid is also used to treat hypothyroidism when your body doesn't make any T4 or T3. The brand Armour Thyroid is an extract from the thyroid gland of pigs. It has both T4 and T3. It is also used to treat goiter and may be used to diagnose a thyroid disorder.

Desiccated thyroid may not be suitable for you in certain circumstances such as if you have thyrotoxicosis or a problem with your adrenal gland that is not controlled with treatment. Your doctor will discuss whether desiccated thyroid is appropriate for you, and its benefits and risks.

Hyperthyroidism

As noted in prior chapters, this is a condition in which the thyroid gland is overactive. Causes may include Graves' disease (an autoimmune condition), toxic multinodular goiter (overactive thyroid nodules), or pituitary gland tumor. In rare cases it may be caused by excess iodine intake.

Symptoms include the following:

- anxiety
- sweating
- irritability, nervousness, restlessness
- racing heart rate
- brittle nails and hair
- bulging eyes (Graves' disease)
- weight loss
- increased appetite

Diagnosis

If T4/thyroxine levels are high and your TSH levels are low in blood tests administered by your physician, that may mean you have an overactive thyroid gland. Your doctor will check for abnormal antibodies if they suspect an autoimmune condition like Graves' disease.

You may also be given a low amount of radioactive iodine (iodine-131 or iodine-123) by injection or take it orally by mouth. This is another way for your doctor to see how much your thyroid gland absorbs and if you have thyroid cancer. If your thyroid takes up a lot of the radioiodine, your thyroid gland is overactive. Most people don't have a reaction to this test. If your doctor orders this type of test, they'll discuss the risks with you.

Iodine contrast dyes have between 140 and 400 mg of iodine in 1 mL of oral or intravenous solution, and they are often used for diagnosing various conditions. Examples of the use of iodine contrast dyes include computed tomography (CT) and angiography.

However, contrast agents containing high amounts of iodine are not recommended for people who have existing thyroid conditions or severe kidney disease. If you have an existing thyroid condition or severe kidney disease, be sure your doctor knows.

Treatment

If you've been diagnosed with hyperthyroidism, the treatment generally depends on the cause. It may involve blocking the thyroid gland from making thyroid hormones or even destroying the thyroid gland. And, if it's caused by excess iodine, correcting iodine levels can help the thyroid gland to work normally again. In some cases, you may need to take medications to correct hyperthyroidism.

Medications

- Methimazole (Tapazole)—Your doctor may prescribe this anti-thyroid medication to stop the thyroid gland from making thyroid hormones. This can resolve hyperthyroid symptoms.
- Propylthiouracil—This medication stops the thyroid gland from producing thyroid hormones.
- Beta blockers—This class of medication is used to control some symptoms of hyperthyroidism such as fast heart rate or sweating.

Your doctor can provide more details about these medications, their uses, their side effects, and much more.

Radioactive Iodine

Radioiodine (iodine-131) is used to treat thyroid cancer (follicular, papillary), other serious thyroid conditions such as goiter, or hyperthyroidism when other treatments are not effective or suitable. Radioiodine is taken up by the thyroid gland and it destroys thyroid tissues and cells, inactivating the gland to stop it from making thyroid hormones. It is taken either as a pill or in liquid form. It's effective for people who have Graves' disease, toxic multinodular goiter, well-differentiated thyroid cancer, or toxic adenoma.[101] After

---

101 Han Shuwen et al., "Nine Genes Mediate the Therapeutic Effects of Iodine-131 Radiotherapy in Thyroid Carcinoma Patients," *Disease Markers* (2020): 9369341, doi:

taking radioiodine, you become hypothyroid and may need to take synthetic thyroid hormone medication daily.

Surgery

Surgery is recommended for some types of thyroid cancer to remove all or part of the thyroid gland. There are several types of thyroid cancer including follicular thyroid cancer, medullary thyroid cancer, papillary thyroid cancer, and thyroid cancer that is of an undetermined type.

The American Thyroid Association guidelines recommend total removal of the thyroid gland for tumors more than 1 centimeter in size, and partial lobe removal for tumors less than or equal to 1 centimeter in size.[102]

In some cases, when surgery doesn't remove all of the cancer, radioiodine (iodine-131) is used after surgery to kill any remaining cancer cells.

After treatment with radioactive iodine, the person is kept in isolation for 48 hours to avoid contact with others. This is because, after treatment with iodine-131, the radioactive iodine that's not absorbed by the thyroid is eliminated through urine, sweat, saliva, and other body fluids. This process may take around a week and may negatively affect people who come in close physical contact with the person who received treatment with radioactive iodine.

Surgery to remove part or all of the thyroid gland makes the person hypothyroid and requires taking synthetic thyroid hormone medication daily since the body stops making it.

10.1155/2020/9369341.

102 Robert C. Smallridge et al., "American Thyroid Association Guidelines for Management of Patients with Anaplastic Thyroid Cancer," *Thyroid* 22, no. 11 (2022): 1104–39, doi: 10.1089/thy.2012.0302.

Thyroid Nodules and Thyroid Cancer

Thyroid nodules are growths on the thyroid gland. They may be solid or filled with fluid. Various factors increase the risk for thyroid nodules, including Hashimoto's thyroiditis, iodine deficiency, and receiving ionizing radiation treatment.[103] Other factors that increase risks include smoking, obesity, alcohol consumption, uterine fibroids, goiter, and other metabolic conditions.

Thyroid nodules are more common in women than men, and in a majority of cases they are benign (noncancerous).[104] However, in a small percentage of cases, thyroid nodules may be cancerous. Cancer is more common in men than in women. Generally, small nodules are not noticeable and don't cause any symptoms. Large nodules can cause goiter, difficulty swallowing or breathing, and pain. Nodules can make your thyroid gland malfunction and become either over- or underactive. This can lead to hyperthyroidism or hypothyroidism.

Thyroid cancer is rare and occurs in only 4 to 6 percent of adults. It is also very rare in children but is more aggressive when it occurs in children. It is the most common type of endocrine cancer in children.[105] In children, it can cause pain, hoarseness, trouble swallowing, and a lump in the neck.

Diagnosis

Since thyroid gland malfunction rarely has symptoms, it is typically diagnosed during other routine checkups. However, if you're experi-

---

103 Edgar A. Zamora, Swapnil Khare, and Sebastiano Cassaro, "Thyroid Nodule," in *StatPearls* (Treasure Island, FL: StatPearls Publishing, 2022).

104 Bryan R. Haugen et al., "2015 American Thyroid Association Management Guidelines for Adult Patients with Thyroid Nodules and Differentiated Thyroid Cancer: The American Thyroid Association Guidelines Task Force on Thyroid Nodules and Differentiated Thyroid Cancer," *Thyroid* 26, no. 1 (2016): 1–133, http://doi.org/10.1089/thy.2015.0020.

105 Vera A. Paulson, Erin R. Rudzinski, and Douglas S. Hawkins, "Thyroid Cancer in the Pediatric Population," *Genes (Basel)* 10 no.9 (2019): 723, doi: 10.3390/genes10090723.

encing changes in your weight, energy levels, temperature sensitivity, or mood, make an appointment to talk with your doctor to get a diagnosis.

If you have a growth or other symptoms, your doctor may order certain tests to confirm the presence of a thyroid nodule.

These tests may include the following:

∝ imaging tests (CT scan, ultrasound, radioiodine test)

∝ thyroid function test (TSH)

∝ biopsy to check for cancer

Treatment

Treatment depends on the test results. If there is no change in thyroid hormones and the nodule is benign, your doctor may just monitor you.

If your thyroid hormones are out of balance, your doctor may prescribe medication such as levothyroxine for hypothyroidism.

Thyroid Cancer Treatment

In a small number of cases, nodules may be cancerous. If you're diagnosed with thyroid cancer, your doctor will discuss your treatment options and what you can expect with treatment.

Treatments may include the following:

∝ surgery to remove the cancer

∝ radioactive iodine after surgery to destroy and inactivate the gland in order to stop new cancer growth

∝ external-beam radiation treatment to kill cancer cells or slow the growth of cancer when the thyroid gland doesn't take up iodine during diagnosis and has spread to other areas of the body (used for anaplastic thyroid cancer and medullary thyroid cancer)[106]

A 2022 study found adults who consumed higher amounts of ultra-processed foods had a higher risk for developing subclinical hyperthyroidism.[107] This is a condition in which the thyroid gland is overactive, but you may not have clinical symptoms. Subclinical hyperthyroidism is also associated with higher heart-related risk factors such as atrial fibrillation (irregular heart rhythm), which can increase the risk for stroke, heart failure, even death.

Your diet is important for a healthy thyroid gland. In chapter 7, we'll talk about how your nutrition is crucial to keeping thyroid hormones balanced, including iodine levels.

Treatments for Iodine Deficiency

There are various types of iodine treatments including radioactive iodine, over-the-counter supplements, and food sources of iodine. It's important to keep in mind that if you have a history of thyroid-related conditions or endemic iodine deficiency, you're more vulnerable to thyroid disorders from iodine-related causes such as taking supplements containing excessive amounts of iodine.

Treatment for iodine deficiency depends on your iodine level and other associated factors.

---

106 American Cancer Society, "External Beam Radiation Therapy for Thyroid Cancer," 2019, https://www.cancer.org/cancer/thyroid-cancer/treating/external-beam-radiation.html.

107 Juanjuan Zhang et al., "Ultra-Processed Food Consumption and the Risk of Subclinical Thyroid Dysfunction: A Prospective Cohort Study," *Food Function* 13, no. 6 (2022): 3431–40, doi: 10.1039/d1fo03279h.

Treatments may include the following:

- $\propto$ increasing dietary iodine
- $\propto$ supplements
- $\propto$ use of iodized salt
- $\propto$ treating thyroid conditions

For mild iodine deficiency, depending on your individual circumstances, your doctor may discuss using iodized salt if you don't have high blood pressure or other reasons to avoid additional salt in your diet. Your doctor may also suggest adding iodine to your diet through certain foods rich in iodine. We'll discuss these in detail in chapter 7.

For moderate or serious iodine deficiency, your treatment depends on your level of deficiency and if you have other health complications. Your doctor may suggest iodine supplements. Since there are many types of supplements, and quality, purity, and potency can vary among products, it's helpful to understand how to choose supplements. We'll go over this in chapter 8.

If you're planning to become pregnant or are breastfeeding, talk with your obstetrician about your iodine levels and needs. They can guide you on whether you need a multivitamin that contains iodine. They can also discuss how to make sure you're getting enough iodine through your diet.

A good tip to estimate your iodine intake is to look at the iodine content of various foods you eat. This can help you gauge if you're likely to be deficient. Talk with your doctor about your diet, particularly if you have a restrictive diet such as a vegan diet or a dairy-free diet.

Newborns are tested for their thyroid function after birth. If they are iodine deficient, they may be given thyroid hormone supplements. In some cases, this may be lifelong, depending on how their thyroid gland is working.

Treatment for Iodine Excess

For most people, it's rare for excess iodine levels to cause serious health problems. However, if you have a history of thyroid disorder or have experienced iodine deficiency in the past, you're more likely to encounter problems, even with small increases in iodine levels.

Treatment for excess iodine levels depends on the level and other factors. Generally, treatments are the opposite of iodine deficiency treatments.

Options can include the following:

- changing your diet to reduce iodine for mild excess (avoid seafood, certain dairy products, seaweed)
- stopping iodine supplements (if you are taking them)
- treating thyroid conditions (hyperthyroidism, hypothyroidism, Graves' disease)
- avoiding iodized salt
- for severe iodine poisoning, taking activated charcoal to stop your body from absorbing excess iodine, implementing supportive measures for breathing difficulties (ventilator), and managing other health conditions

If you've developed mild hypothyroidism from taking too much iodine, your doctor may recommend lowering your dietary iodine levels. In some cases, this is all that's needed to correct the problem. However, if it's more serious, your doctor may prescribe thyroid hormones to regulate your thyroid gland. Some people will need to take these long term.

As noted earlier, if you have Graves' disease, your doctor may recommend anti-thyroid medications such as methimazole or propylthiouracil, radioactive iodine treatment, or thyroid surgery. Your treatment depends on the severity of your condition. Your doctor will discuss all your available treatment options based on your individual situation.

Iodine is an important micronutrient that's vital for our bodies. You'll find plenty of experts touting the benefits of supplementing with iodine. But remember, taking too much iodine can have negative consequences. This is especially true if you have a history of thyroid problems. Before deciding to supplement with iodine, check with your doctor. They can explain the benefits and risks of taking iodine based on your individual health history. After all, you wouldn't want to unknowingly worsen your thyroid health.

CHAPTER 7

Dietary Sources of Iodine

As you've learned so far, it's crucial to have adequate iodine levels for your thyroid gland to work properly in order to make thyroid hormones. And thyroid hormones regulate many important functions in your body: your brain, your energy level, your temperature, and so much more.

Iodine and selenium are important micronutrients that can affect thyroid-stimulating antibodies and thyroid function. Deficiencies in these nutrients can cause or alter the course of autoimmune-generated thyroid problems such as Graves' disease.

The main way your body gets iodine is through dietary sources. The common forms include iodide, iodate, or organically bound iodine. Even though your thyroid gland needs just a small amount to work normally, if you're consistently not getting enough iodine through the foods you eat daily, eventually you'll become iodine deficient. On the other hand, if you're regularly consuming foods that are very high in iodine, you're at greater risk for developing iodine excess.

As we've discussed previously, both low and high iodine levels can alter how the thyroid gland works, causing an imbalance of thyroid hormones and related conditions such as hypothyroidism or hyper-thyroidism, nodules, or goiter.

The most common sources of daily iodine intake for individuals are iodized salt, dairy, bread, and certain types of seafood.

You might wonder, since iodized salt has been around nearly a hundred years and most households have access to this everyday staple, why does iodine deficiency still exist around the world?

We've touched on a few reasons for iodine deficiency such as lack of access to nutritious food sources, poor soil and water conditions, avoidance of salt due to health reasons, or following a restricted diet.

Knowing and understanding dietary sources of iodine, and taking a look at your personal diet and what you eat on a regular basis, will help you determine whether you're getting sufficient iodine or if you need to adjust your food intake.

Recommended Dietary Allowance

One of the challenges with estimating iodine sufficiency for populations and individuals is the different definitions and guidelines used to define iodine adequacy. Some scientists propose using the average requirement (AR) to estimate iodine adequacy for populations.[108] AR is defined as the average daily iodine consumption projected to meet the needs of 50 percent of healthy individuals at a particular life stage. On the other hand, average intake and RDA guidelines are defined as the average daily level estimated to meet the iodine requirements for almost all (98 percent of) healthy individuals.[109] These differences in defining iodine levels for populations and individuals can cause confusion and misinterpretation of data in determining iodine sufficiency.

As we've mentioned previously, in certain times of your life, your body's need for iodine increases, and if your diet isn't a good source of iodine, you can become deficient. Also, if your diet doesn't include

108 Maria Andersson and Christian P. Braegger, "The Role of Iodine for Thyroid Function in Lactating Women and Infants," *Endocrine Reviews* 43, no. 3 (2022): 469–506, doi: 10.1210/endrev/bnab029.

109 Christine Baumgartner et al., "Thyroid Function Within the Normal Range, Subclinical Hypothyroidism, and the Risk of Atrial Fibrillation," *Circulation* 136, no. 22 (2017): 2100–16, doi: 10.1161/CIRCULATIONAHA.117.028753.

iodized salt or the other common sources of iodine (dairy, seafood, bread), you have a higher risk for becoming deficient.

The US RDA for iodine is 150 mcg per day for adults. It's higher for pregnant women (220 mcg) and breastfeeding women (290 mcg). However, there are some problems in estimating how much iodine you're actually getting through your diet based on the foods you eat daily. This is one of the challenges surrounding iodine and the RDA guidelines, and why many people around the world may be mildly iodine deficient without being aware of it.

One of the reasons it's difficult to estimate iodine content of foods in the US is because not all foods have iodine amounts listed. The United States doesn't require iodine nutritional content to be listed in food products. In fact, the US Department of Agriculture (USDA) didn't begin listing iodine in its nutrient database until 2019. You can enter various foods in the USDA's FoodData Central search and learn more about nutrient content.[110]

The other reason it's difficult to estimate average daily intake of iodine is that, according to research, the iodine content of foods can vary. This can make it difficult to learn whether you're at adequate levels, in deficiency, or in excess according to your dietary habits. Scientists believe some possible reasons for variations in iodine levels in foods from time to time might be due to different farming techniques or processing methods, seasonal changes, where food is grown, and even food is cooked. For example, if you recall, boiling certain types of high-iodine-containing seaweed can lower its iodine level markedly (up to 99%).

While the lack of iodine nutritional information can present challenges in calculating your daily iodine intake, as long as you're not on a very restrictive diet, you should be getting adequate amounts of it.

110   Go to https://fdc.nal.usda.gov/ to try out the USDA's FoodCentral search.

The key to iodine balance is making sure you're eating a well-rounded diet containing iodine from a variety of food sources. As noted, vegetables and fruits are not a good source of iodine because they contain minimal amounts.

If you're on a restrictive diet, you may need to supplement with iodine to make sure you're not deficient. We'll talk about available iodine supplements, and how to choose from the many products, in chapter 8.

Iodine Content of Various Types of Food

Iodine added to any food in the United States is considered a food additive.[111] The label has to list the percent Daily Value (DV) of iodine in the food. However, this doesn't apply to dietary supplements. The FDA loosely regulates dietary supplement ingredient standards.

Dairy products provide some of the highest sources of iodine.[112] It is estimated that between 13 and 64 percent of our iodine needs are met by dairy products.[113] In the US, they account for an estimated 50 percent of total iodine intake. In fact, one serving of milk can provide up to 57 percent of a daily serving of iodine. However, there is wide variability in iodine content in different milk products. Again, this makes it hard to figure out your daily levels, especially if you're vulnerable to thyroid conditions.

111 P. R. Trumbo, "FDA Regulations Regarding Iodine Addition to Foods and Labeling of Foods Containing Added Iodine," *American Journal of Clinical Nutrition* 104, supplement no. 3 (2016): 864S–67S, doi: 10.3945/ajcn.115.110338.

112 Janet M. Roseland et al., "USDA, FDA, and ODS-NIH Database for the Iodine Content of Common Foods," (2022), https://www.ars.usda.gov/ARSUSERFILES /80400535/DATA/IODINE/IODINE%20DATABASE_RELEASE_2_DOCUMENTATION.PDF.

113 Olivia L. van de Reijden, Michael B. Zimmermann, and Valeria Galetti, "Iodine in Dairy Milk: Sources, Concentrations and Importance to Human Health," *Best Practice & Research Clinical Endocrinology & Metabolism* 31, no. 4 (2017): 385–95, doi: 10.1016/j .beem.2017.10.004; Janet M. Roseland et al., "Large Variability of Iodine Content in Retail Cow's Milk in the U.S.," *Nutrients* 12, no. 5 (2020): 1246, doi: 10.3390/nu12051246.

Food Groups and Iodine Content

Food Group	Iodine Content
Dairy	Plain Greek yogurt 51 mcg
Eggs	Whole dried egg 274 mcg; dried yolk 349 mcg; raw egg yolk 177 mcg
Vegetables	Miscellaneous <10 mcg
Fruits	Miscellaneous <5 mcg
Seafood	Lobster 185 mcg; mollusk 104 mcg; haddock 227 mcg
Meat	Chicken or beef <5 mcg
Grains	Pasta boiled with iodized salt 29 mcg
Seaweed	Dried nori 2,320 mcg
Fast Food	Cheeseburger w/ iodate dough conditioner 278 mcg; egg +cheese + ham Muffin 25 mcg
Baked Goods	White bread roll with iodate dough conditioner 1,196 mcg; Sliced white bread with iodate dough conditioner 693 mcg

Factors that can cause alterations to iodine content of foods include the following:

∝ iodine-based milk sanitation techniques used by dairies

∝ animals eating goitrogenic foods[114]

∝ where animals graze (pasture soil versus sea area)

∝ any iodine supplementation of animals

∝ the season (iodine concentration in store-bought milk is higher in winter than summer)

---

114 W. P. Weiss et al., "Effect of Including Canola Meal and Supplemental Iodine in Diets of Dairy Cows on Short-Term Changes in Iodine Concentrations in Milk," *Journal of Dairy Science* 98, no. 7 (2015): 4841–49, doi: 10.3168/jds.2014-9209.

For example, in one study, cows that were fed a canola-meal diet had the lowest iodine levels compared with cows that were given other types of feed and cows that were given iodine supplements. Although the amount of supplemental iodine given to dairy cows is regulated in the US, food-based iodine factors are not regulated and contribute to variations in iodine in dairy products.

A 2022 Total Diet Study nutrition report analyzing data on nutrients and contaminants in foods in the US from 2018–2020 by the US Department of Agriculture done in partnership with several other US government agencies, including the National Institutes of Health Office of Dietary Supplements and the US Food and Drug Administration Center for Food Safety and Applied Nutrition, provides a detailed list of the nutrient content of various foods. Researchers are currently analyzing the data to learn more about micronutrients such as iodine to determine if there have been changes from the past.

If you recall, studies based on the NHANES surveys found increasing iodine deficiency over the time period studied. Studies have also shown that women of reproductive age, Black Americans, and young adults are mildly iodine deficient.[115]

It is hoped that the Total Diet Study report analysis will provide new information about food sources of iodine and whether the US is still at adequate levels for the majority of the population.

Goitrogenic Foods

As noted in chapter 3, the term goitrogens means substances, including foods that can cause goiter, or swelling of the thyroid gland. Goitrogenic foods can block the amount of iodine your thyroid gland can access, and they can also obstruct other elements needed for

---

115 Kyun Won Lee et al., "Changes in Iodine Status Among US Adults, 2001–2012," *International Journal of Food Sciences and Nutrition* 67, no. 2 (2016): 184–94, doi: 10.3109/09637486.2016.1144717.

normal thyroid hormone production. For most people, goitrogens don't pose problems with thyroid function. In rare cases, eating excessive amounts of goitrogenic foods regularly may increase the risk for developing iodine deficiency and thyroid problems.

Goitrogenic foods include cruciferous vegetables such as cauliflower, broccoli, brussels sprouts, collard greens, kale, and others in the *Brassica* family of foods. One benefit of cruciferous vegetables is their anticancer properties. Soy products also contain isoflavones, which can block thyroid hormone production.

Cruciferous vegetables are rich in antioxidants and fiber. These compounds have been shown to have anticancer properties.[116] Most types of cruciferous vegetables have low levels of goitrogens, but brussels sprouts, collard greens, and some species of Russian kale have higher levels of goitrogens.

Currently, few studies exist that report a link between thyroid disorder and eating goitrogenic vegetables. One Chinese study from 2010 described an 88-year-old Chinese woman who developed myxedema coma after eating 1 to 1.5 kilograms of raw bok choy daily for several months.[117] This seems to be an extreme and isolated case since no other such reports are available in the literature.

Myxedema coma is caused by severe advanced hypothyroidism as a result of inadequate thyroid hormone production. It can cause slow heart rate, slow breathing, shock, and, ultimately, coma. It can include skin changes such as swelling of the face, eyes, lips, tongue,

116 Peter Felker, Ronald Bunch, and Angela M. Leung, "Concentrations of Thiocyanate and Goitrin in Human Plasma, Their Precursor Concentrations in Brassica Vegetables, and Associated Potential Risk for Hypothyroidism," *Nutrition Reviews* 74, no. 4 (2016): 248–58, doi: 10.1093/nutrit/nuv110; Ahmad Faizal Abdull Razis and Noramaliza Mohd Noor, "Cruciferous Vegetables: Dietary Phytochemicals for Cancer Prevention," *Asian Pacific Journal of Cancer Prevention* 14, no. 3 (2013): 1565–70, doi: 10.7314/apjcp.2013.14.3.1565; Michael Kob, "Cruciferous Vegetables and the Thyroid Gland: Friends or Foes?" *Complementary Medical Research* 25, no. 1 (2018), doi: 10.1159/000488417.

117 Michael Chu and Terry F. Seltzer, "Myxedema Coma Induced by Ingestion of Raw Bok Choy," *The New England Journal of Medicine* 362, no. 20 (2010): 1945–6, doi: 10.1056/NEJMc0911005.

and skin. Myxedema coma is also referred to as myxedema crisis and is considered a medical emergency.

If you have an existing thyroid disorder, or are moderately or severely iodine deficient, it's a good idea to discuss your diet and consumption of goitrogenic vegetables with your doctor. So far there are no data that show eating a healthy diet, including some cruciferous vegetables, poses a problem for thyroid function. Boiling or cooking cruciferous vegetables also lowers goitrogenic compounds.

Diets high in soy products such as tofu, tempeh, soy milk, or miso have some health benefits. Studies have shown consuming soy products may lower total cholesterol and LDL cholesterol to a small extent. Soy may modestly lower hot flashes associated with menopause for some women, and possibly lower blood pressure and breast cancer risk.[118] However, much is still unknown regarding the possible effects of consuming soy products for people with thyroid problems, including those who may be iodine deficient. Infants born with hypothyroidism who are prescribed levothyroxine and are drinking a soy-based formula may need adjustments to their levothyroxine dose to manage hypothyroidism.

If you have normal thyroid function, eating a balanced diet including some soy-based products does not pose thyroid-related health risks. And if you have a thyroid disorder and take medication, as long as you're not consuming excessive amounts of soy, generally soy doesn't cause health issues. However, always check with your doctor about your soy consumption and any concerns. Heating, soaking, and fermentation of soy products such as tofu may also lower their goitrogenic properties.

118 Christopher R. D'Adam and Azieie Sahin, "Soy Foods and Supplementation: A Review of Commonly Perceived Health Benefits and Risks," *Alternative Therapies in Health and Medicine* 20, no. 1 (2014): 39–51, PMID: 24473985.

High-Iodine Foods

As we've discussed, generally, foods that are high in iodine include dairy products, grain, certain types of seafood, and seaweed. Most people who consume a varied diet that has a balance of different categories of food sources get adequate amounts of iodine through their diet.

According to data from the 2022 Total Diet Study report, the following are examples of foods with high iodine content. Fruits and vegetables are noticeably missing from the high-iodine food chart that follows because they have negligible amounts of iodine. This chart can be helpful to evaluate diet patterns and iodine intake. Again, keep in mind that these values are estimates of high-iodine-content foods, and assigned iodine values can change based on season, preservatives, processing techniques used, and more.

Examples of High-Iodine-Content Foods
from FDA Total Diet Study 2018–2020[119]

Meat/Poultry/Fish/Eggs

Frozen fish sticks / fish patty	507 mcg
Baked cod fish	1,696 mcg
Frankfurter (beef or beef + pork)	533 mcg
Hard-boiled eggs	673 mcg
Lunch meat (bologna)	187 mcg
Pre-cooked shrimp	141 mcg
Salmon	122 mcg
Canned tuna	106 mcg
Dried salami	97 mcg
Canned clam chowder	109 mcg

Other Foods

Veggie burger	95 mcg
Fruit Popsicle	2,268 mcg
Milk chocolate candy bar	433 mcg
Protein powder	977 mcg
Grapefruit juice	157 mcg
Pumpkin pie	277 mcg

---

119 The latest FDA Total Diet Study was published in 2022 (FDA.gov/media/159751
/download) and is based on data from 2018–2020.

⚖ The **Iodine Balancing** Handbook

Examples of High-Iodine-Content Foods
from FDA Total Diet Study 2018–2020

Dairy

Whole milk	300 mcg
Low-fat yogurt	270 mcg
Cream cheese	240 mcg
Monterey Jack cheese	413 mcg
American processed cheese	457 mcg
Mozzarella cheese	500 mcg
Reduced-fat cottage cheese	423 mcg
Sour cream	290 mcg
Swiss cheese	1,505 mcg
Half-and-half cream	296 mcg
Vanilla milkshake	360 mcg

Bread

Pre-sliced white bread	2,674 mcg
Pre-sliced whole wheat bread	1,282 mcg
Bread crumbs	1,117 mcg
Hamburger/hot dog bun	4,034 mcg
Homemade cornbread	383 mcg

As we've mentioned previously, it can be difficult to measure iodine content of foods accurately because levels can change for various reasons. Further, there is a lack of clearly defined criteria for what are considered optimal iodine levels for groups that need higher levels such as pregnant or breastfeeding women. Relying solely on nutrient content surveys of iodine concentration in various foods may generate assessment gaps in determining iodine sufficiency for vulnerable populations.

Food-nutrient content analysis has limitations and may not be sufficient if used alone to assess iodine malnutrition in vulnerable populations. Further, having more detailed explanations about data collection methods, and possible reasons for shifts in levels, may help raise awareness regarding reasons for potential discrepancies in assigned values.

Consuming a balanced diet with enough of these iodine-rich sources of food helps to keep you in iodine sufficiency. If you don't think you're getting enough iodine from your diet, or have symptoms of iodine deficiency, talk with your doctor. They can check your iodine level and thyroid function.

FDA's Total Diet Study report found foods that were high in iodine included certain types of bread such as white bread, hamburger and hot dog buns (white), and whole wheat bread. Researchers believe this may possibly be due to iodine-based dough conditioners added to bread dough for some product samples. The report also found fruit-flavored Popsicles had a high iodine concentration. They believe this may be due to the addition of FD&C Red #3 food dye, which contains iodine.

You can see from these examples that iodine may be found in unexpected foods due to processing or iodine being added as a supplement to animal diet, sanitation processes, and other factors.[120]

120 Food and Drug Administration, "FDA Total Diet Study (TDS)," FDA.gov, last updated July 15, 2022, https://www.fda.gov/food/science-research-food/total-diet-study; Abby G. Ershow et al., "Development of Databases on Iodine in Foods and Dietary Supplements," Nutrients 10, no. 1 (2018): 100, doi: 10.3390/nu10010100.

⚖️ The **Iodine Balancing** Handbook

Higher Needs with Special Diets

Most people who eat a balanced diet consisting of a variety of different foods have adequate iodine levels. However, if you have special dietary requirements, which don't include many iodine-rich foods, you may be at higher risk for iodine deficiency.

As an example, you might be at risk for iodine deficiency if you avoid these categories of foods:

- dairy
- grains
- seafood
- meats/poultry/eggs

Since being vegan or vegetarian is common today, it's important to be aware of iodine content of various foods to ensure you're getting adequate amounts to remain iodine sufficient.

While few studies have assessed the impact of iodine levels on those who follow special diets, a few older studies have reported that vegans and vegetarians have lower iodine levels than those who eat more varied foods including meats, fish, and eggs.[121]

A 2020 review of studies including over 127,000 people from industrialized countries found those following vegan diets had the lowest iodine concentrations, followed by vegetarians. The study reported individuals following a vegan diet were more often mildly or moderately iodine deficient compared with other groups based on the WHO 150 mcg/day recommended daily intake. The majority of vegans and vegetarians didn't meet adequate iodine concentrations compared with a majority (83 percent) of omnivores.[122]

121 Victor R. Preedy, Gerard N. Burrow, Ronald Watson (Eds.), *Comprehensive Handbook of Iodine: Nutritional, Biochemical, Pathological and Therapeutic Aspects.* (Cambridge, MA: Academic Press, 2009); M Krajcovicová-Kudláčková et al., "Iodine Deficiency in Vegetarians and Vegans," *Annals of Nutrition and Metabolism* 47, no. 5 (2003): 183–5, doi: 10.1159/000070483.

122 Elizabeth R. Eveleigh et al., "Vegans, Vegetarians, and Omnivores: How Does Dietary Choice Influence Iodine Intake? A Systematic Review," *Nutrients* 12, no. 6 (May

Vegans, who eliminate dairy, meat, fish, and eggs, are at higher risk for developing iodine deficiency.[123] Another study found that people who followed a lacto-ovo-vegetarian lifestyle were 9 percent more likely to have hypothyroidism than those who followed a mixed diet.

Further, consuming alternative nondairy-based milk and nonfortified-plant-based meals increases the vulnerability for iodine deficiency. This is particularly true for people living in countries that already have higher rates of iodine deficiency.

Manufacturers of alternative dairy products (soy, almond, etc.) and plant-based foods should indicate iodine content on the labels to help identify iodine sources of these types of foods.

If you follow a vegan diet, you may need to include alternative iodine-rich sources or use iodine supplements to stay at adequate levels. Keep in mind that eating too much seaweed, which is high in iodine, or taking certain iodine supplements with undisclosed amounts of iodine can also pose problems of developing iodine excess or heavy metal exposure due to contamination.

Studies have shown that iron and selenium, in addition to iodine, play an important role in normal thyroid function.[124] If you're a vegan or vegetarian, ensuring you're getting sufficient amounts of these three nutrients is crucial for normal thyroid regulation. Studies have also shown that having adequate selenium and iodine levels may provide protective benefits against autoimmune thyroiditis.[125]

2020): 1606, doi: 10.3390/nu12061606.

123 Martin Světnička and Eva El-Lababidi, "Problematics of Iodine Saturation Among Children on the Vegan Diet," *Casopis Lékaru Ceských (Journal of Czech Physicians)* 160, no. 6 (2021): 237–41, English, PMID: 35045716.

124 Margaret P. Rayman, "Multiple Nutritional Factors and Thyroid Disease, with Particular Reference to Autoimmune Thyroid Disease," *The Proceedings of Nutrition Society* 78, no. 1 (2019): 34–44, doi: 10.1017/S0029665118001192.

125 Edoardo Guastamacchia et al., "Selenium and Iodine in Autoimmune Thyroiditis," *Endocrine, Metabolic & Immune Disorders Drug Targets* 15, no. 4 (2015): 288–92, doi: 10.2174/1871530315666150619094242.

Increasingly, vegetarian and vegan diets are popular. Since fruits and vegetables are low in iodine content, it's important to substitute enough iodine-rich foods to stay at healthy iodine levels. Infants and growing children need adequate iodine levels for proper growth and development and to maintain healthy thyroid function and avoid thyroid conditions from long-term iodine deficiency.

If you follow a specific diet, see the "Helpful Resources" chapter for a listing of various dietary professional organizations. You can reach out to them for help in locating someone where you live who can help you develop a food source guide to stay iodine balanced.

CHAPTER 8

Who Needs Iodine Supplements?

Whether you need iodine supplements is based on your iodine levels, your symptoms, other health conditions you may have, and other factors that must be considered (such as pregnancy). As we've discussed, iodine deficiency can cause hypothyroidism and subsequently permanent brain and physical developmental disabilities in fetuses and infants. Iodine deficiency is believed to be the most common cause of preventable brain abnormalities around the world.

As we've discussed throughout this book, individuals who may need supplements include the following:

- pregnant and nursing women who are deficient (based on physician's counsel)
- vegans or vegetarians who are deficient
- others who live in areas with endemic iodine deficiency
- those who don't have access to iodized salt and are iodine deficient

Most people can meet their daily iodine needs through the use of common iodized salt in combination with iodine-rich foods, as we detailed in the previous chapter. But if you don't consume enough of these, you may need an iodine supplement based on your specific circumstances.

Typically, if you're experiencing symptoms of iodine deficiency or your doctor suspects a thyroid disorder, they'll order tests to check your iodine and thyroid hormone levels.

Depending on the severity of your deficiency, your doctor may recommend you talk with a dietitian or nutritionist to boost dietary iodine intake naturally.

However, if your doctor feels your deficiency is more serious, they may recommend that you take iodine supplements. They'll suggest a dosage and recommend the type of iodine best for you. Your doctor will also regularly monitor your iodine and thyroid hormone levels while you're taking iodine supplements.

Types of Supplements

There is a lot to understand about dietary supplements and their benefits and risks before buying iodine.

First, there are hundreds of different sources and types of iodine supplements available. And they contain vastly different amounts of iodine which can impact your thyroid health. Remember, iodine excess is just as harmful to your health as iodine deficiency. Not knowing how much you're taking can increase your risk of getting too much iodine.

The FDA requires food additives and nutrient ingredients added to foods or supplements to be listed on the product labeling. For example, if cuprous (copper) iodide or potassium iodide is added to salt, the label must read as follows: "This salt supplies iodide, a necessary nutrient." However, currently there are no regulations that oversee ingredient standards for dietary supplements. The FDA doesn't regulate iodine fortification of foods or supplements. So, multivitamins are not required to include iodine. But if iodine is added to a supplement, it has to be noted on the label.

According to FDA regulations for dietary supplement labeling standards, supplement labels must have the following:

∝ product name
∝ labeling facts (ingredient listing and amounts)

- quantity of contents
- inactive ingredients (these are ingredients such as binders and fillers that don't affect how the supplement works)
- name and address of manufacturer, distributor, and packer

There are all kinds of iodine supplements, such as tablets, gummies, capsules, and liquids, which have different types and amounts of iodine. The amount of iodine, ingredient source, cost, and quality can vary among available products. Products may also contain other ingredients to "boost" thyroid function such as tyrosine (amino acid) or selenium (micronutrient). Some products marketed as prenatal support have other vitamins and minerals in addition to iodine.

Strengths can vary from as low as 225 mcg, which provides 150 percent of the recommended daily intake (RDI), to over 12,000 mcg, which is over 8,000 percent of RDI.

The American Thyroid Association guidelines suggest avoiding supplements that contain more than 500 mcg per day of iodine.

This is why it's important to talk with your doctor or pharmacist before purchasing any dietary supplements. They can guide you to the appropriate supplement based on your iodine and thyroid hormone levels.

Examples of types of iodine supplements include the following:

- potassium iodide
- sodium iodide
- kelp-derived iodine
- spirulina-based iodine
- prenatal vitamins with iodine

There are numerous brands with different iodine-based products available online and through health food stores, pharmacies, and other retail stores.

Quality Matters

Dietary supplement sales have been growing globally for well over a decade. According to recent estimates, global sales in 2019 were nearly $353 billion USD. There are many products, and in the US, the FDA only loosely regulates them. This can make it hard to select quality supplements.

Also, keep in mind that "natural" doesn't mean safe or effective. Many dietary supplement and nutraceutical products sold online and on store shelves contain unsafe amounts of contaminants such as lead, mercury, and other harmful undisclosed products. This can be dangerous if contaminants build up in the body over time.

One important tip is to look for purity and potency standards on the label. Choose reputable brands. Generally, products that are tested and verified by independent third-party laboratories are more likely to have quality ingredients in the amounts listed on the label.

Healthcare Professional Guidance

It can be overwhelming to see the number of iodine supplements available over the counter and online. This can make it difficult to decide which one is best. Product quality standards can also differ greatly between manufacturers. For example, many products may not contain the amount listed on the label (higher or lower amounts).

This is why your local community pharmacist is a great resource. If your doctor suggests taking an iodine supplement, they can guide you to quality products. Letting your pharmacist know about dietary supplements you're taking can also prevent drug interactions with your other prescription medications.

You can schedule a time to sit down and talk with the pharmacist about all your medications and over-the-counter products to make sure they are safe and effective and don't interact with your other medications.

CHAPTER 9

Final Points

Based on all the benefits of iodine we've outlined, this micronutrient is significant for normal body function. So, is it time to go out and get some iodine supplements? Not quite. As exciting as the research is about the many potential benefits of iodine, there is still a great deal to understand about its effectiveness, dosage, and safety.

If you've turned to this book, you've clearly wanted to learn more about iodine and how it affects your health. There is a lot of information about iodine on the web and in books. Some online forums, blogs, and books suggest we're getting too much iodine and it's causing numerous health issues. Many other books and websites propose we're suffering from iodine deficiency. Which is true? The facts are less dramatic.

Let's look at some facts to help navigate the iodine discussion:

- Most of us get enough iodine from our regular diet to maintain adequate levels.
- Those on restrictive diets are more susceptible to iodine deficiencies and thyroid-related conditions.
- Iodine levels have been going down in the US over the past several years.
- Both low and high levels of iodine can cause health problems in the long term.
- Iodine deficiency is more common in resource-poor areas due to lack of access to high-quality food or water and also due to poor soil conditions.
- Individual iodine testing procedures are often inaccurate.
- Pregnant and breastfeeding women require more iodine to support themselves and their developing babies.

- Many obstetricians and midwives don't discuss iodine levels with their patients.
- Consistently consuming highly goitrogenic (iodine-blocking) foods can lower iodine levels in the long term.
- People with thyroid conditions are more sensitive to changes in iodine levels (up or down).
- Iodine poisoning is rare but can pose a life-threatening medical crisis that needs immediate medical attention.
- Iodine supplements can vary widely in their levels of iodine and their quality.
- Iodine supplements can interact with other medications.
- Scientists are still discovering the benefits and risks of iodine, its appropriate dosages, and its effectiveness.

Even if you have some of the symptoms of iodine deficiency, don't start taking a supplement without checking with your doctor first. Common symptoms such as weight gain, excessive tiredness, or memory problems may be due to many different health disorders and not necessarily iodine deficiency.

Dietary supplements can also interact with medications. It's always helpful to ask a doctor for their guidance before supplementing. They can discuss your overall health and order appropriate diagnostic tests. This includes checking your iodine and thyroid hormone levels.

According to different researchers, ideal iodine levels for people of various ages are not known. It is also difficult to estimate iodine intake because it's hard to calculate the iodine content of foods accurately. So, your diet is at the heart of iodine balance. What you eat on a regular basis can set you up to have ideal levels or push you into either deficiency or excess.

Health professionals and the international health community also don't agree on appropriate levels. In addition, there is great debate within the medical and scientific communities regarding the established recommended daily allowance for dietary iodine.

Many feel the current adult RDA of 150 mcg per day was provided as a baseline level to prevent goiter, and is not an appropriate level for ideal iodine balance to allow for its full range of benefits. But it's important to know that there are continuous nutrition-monitoring programs and surveys done by various governmental agencies like the United States Department of Agriculture to assess population-level nutritional status. And currently, the majority of people in the US are not considered iodine deficient.

While it's true this provides an overall picture of the population and doesn't address individual factors or health disparities that might contribute to low iodine levels, it still provides signaling on where the US population stands on nutritional status.

The FDA has recently (2022) released a new Total Diet Study report. The report examines nutritional food content from 2018 through 2020. As of the writing of this book, analysis of various nutrients to determine if the US population is meeting average requirements is still ongoing.

This analysis will be an important signal to better understand whether iodine levels are holding steady or declining compared with the last survey. If you're reading this book, you're clearly interested in understanding how iodine affects your health. So be sure to check the FDA-TDS site for updates on iodine analysis.

Some advocates of iodine also argue that the recommended upper limits set for dietary iodine are too conservative. If you recall, levels higher than 300 mcg/L in adults and 500mcg/L in pregnant women are considered excessive, with the maximum level as 1,100 mcg in adults. Research on various dosages of iodine supplements has been inconclusive regarding benefits and risks with higher doses.

This dosage can depend on individual factors not captured in research studies. However, the majority of people without thyroid disorders or other serious health conditions, such as severe kidney disease, tolerate higher doses of iodine without serious harmful effects. But keep in mind that pregnant women and newborns are especially sensitive to high iodine levels and its effects on thyroid function and need closer monitoring to avoid deficiencies or excess.

Iodine continues to remain controversial as a vital nutrient around the world. There are different schools of thought from various scientific, clinical, and functional medicine experts that confuse consumers about their iodine health.

So, what should you take away from reading this book on iodine balance?

The main points to keep in mind are that if you eat a well-balanced diet and include iodized salt as part of your regular diet, you're likely iodine sufficient.

However, if you follow a vegan or vegetarian diet and avoid common sources of iodine-rich foods, you may want to get your iodine and thyroid levels tested with your doctor. Also, if you're experiencing symptoms of thyroid disorder (weight gain, fatigue, temperature sensitivity, etc.) it may help to get your thyroid levels checked.

Your doctor can discuss your risks for iodine deficiency based on your regular diet and suggest whether getting tested makes sense for you.

Once you've been tested, depending on your levels, your doctor will recommend the appropriate next steps. If you're mildly deficient, they may ask you to increase dietary sources of iodine. For serious thyroid health disorders, you may require prescription medications to get your thyroid hormones in check.

There are several wonderful food source databases that list the iodine content of various foods. These databases are included in chapter 10, "Helpful Resources," to help you browse and learn about the nutrient contents of different foods you eat daily.

Take a careful look at your diet, and if you feel you may be low on iodine, talk with your doctor to learn more and take steps to balance your iodine levels.

Helpful Resources

American Academy of Ophthalmology—Thyroid eye disease (www.aao.org/thyroid-eye-disease-resources)

American Cancer Society—Thyroid cancer (www.cancer.org/cancer/thyroid-cancer.html)

American Thyroid Association—Patient resources (www.thyroid.org/patient-thyroid-information)

Asian Americans and Pacific Islanders Academy of Nutrition and Dietetics (AAPIAND)—Food and nutrition resources for AAPI populations (www.aapimig.org/home)

CDC—Micronutrient facts (www.cdc.gov/nutrition/micronutrient-malnutrition/micronutrients)

Centers for Disease Control and Prevention (CDC)—Iodine and breastfeeding (www.cdc.gov/breastfeeding/breastfeeding-special-circumstances/diet-and-micronutrients/iodine.html)

Dietary Guidelines for Americans, 2020-2025—US Department of Agriculture and US Department of Health and Human Services, Ninth Edition, December 2020 (www.dietaryguidelines.gov/resources/2020-2025-dietary-guidelines-online-materials)

FDA—Advice on eating fish (www.fda.gov/food/consumers/advice-about-eating-fish)

FDA's Center for Food Safety and Applied Nutrition Education Resource Library (www.fda.gov/food/resources-you-food/cfsan-education-resource-library)

FDA's Center for Food Safety and Applied Nutrition—Healthy eating index (www.fns.usda.gov/healthy-eating-index-hei)

FDA—Dietary supplements (www.fda.gov/consumers/consumer
-updates/dietary-supplements)

FDA Total Diet Study Report based on FDA monitoring nutrient and
contaminants in foods consumed in the US (www.fda.gov/media
/159745/download)

FDA Total Diet Study Data on food nutrient and contaminants in the
US (www.fda.gov/food/science-research-food/fda-total-diet-study
-tds)

Graves' Disease and Thyroid Foundation—This foundation provides
information and support for Graves' disease and other thyroid
conditions. (https://gdatf.org)

Growing Resilience in the South (GRITS)—A nonprofit providing
free nutritional counseling for vulnerable groups and professional
nutrition programs to raise awareness of African American cultural
influences on foods. (https://gritsinc.org)

Harvard T. H. Chan School of Public Health—Information on iodine
(www.hsph.harvard.edu/nutritionsource/iodine)

The Iodine Global Network—A nonprofit focused on preventing
iodine deficiency around the world. The organization works with
multiple stakeholders (public and private entities, scientific
community, consumers) to raise awareness and find solutions to
eliminate iodine deficiency disorders. (www.ign.org/home.htm)

Latinos and Hispanics in Dietetics and Nutrition, LAHIDAN—
Organization focused on providing diet, nutrition, and health
support for Latino and Hispanic families (www.eatrightlahidan.org
/home)

Light of Life Foundation—This organization provides helpful
information for people diagnosed with thyroid cancer. (https://
lightoflifefoundation.org)

Linus Pauling Institute—Oregon State University, Iodine related
information (https://lpi.oregonstate.edu/mic/minerals/iodine)

Linus Pauling Institute—Oregon State University Micronutrient Information Center, Information on common nutrients (https://lpi .oregonstate.edu/mic/nutrient-index)

National Academies—Summary Report of the Dietary Reference Intakes. (www.nationalacademies.org/our-work/summary-report-of -the-dietary-reference-intakes)

National Institute of Diabetes and Digestive and Kidney Diseases— Information on hyperthyroidism (www.niddk.nih.gov/health -information/endocrine-diseases/hyperthyroidism)

National Institute of Diabetes and Digestive and Kidney Diseases (NIDDK)—Information on hypothyroidism (www.niddk.nih.gov/health -information/endocrine-diseases/hypothyroidism)

National Institutes of Health (NIH)—A great resource covering the importance of iodine for your health (https://ods.od.nih.gov /factsheets/iodine-consumer)

National Institutes of Health Office of Dietary Supplements— Information and latest news on dietary supplements (https://ods .od.nih.gov/index.aspx)

The National Library of Medicine Table of Goitrogenic Foods— Information on iodine deficiency disorders (www.ncbi.nlm.nih.gov /boos/NBK285556/table)

National Organization of Blacks in Dietetics and Nutrition, NOBIDAN— A professional development and support organization for African American dieticians and nutritionists (www.nobidan.org /home)

Thyroid Disease Resource Center— Information resources for thyroid conditions (https://pro.aace.com/disease-state-resources /thyroid)

USDA Agricultural Research Service—Food databases (www.ars .usda.gov/northeast-area/beltsville-md-bhnrc/beltsville-human -nutrition-research-center/methods-and-application-of-food -composition-laboratory/mafcl-site-pages/database-resources)

US Department of Agriculture—Eating healthy on a budget (www .myplate.gov/eat-healthy/healthy-eating-budget)

US Department of Agriculture—Learn about nutrition content of various foods and food sources. (https://fdc.nal.usda.gov)

US Food and Drug Administration—How to understand the nutrition facts label (www.fda.gov/food/new-nutrition-facts-label/how -understand-and-use-nutrition-facts-label)

Acknowledgments

To my husband Koustuv: thank you for always supporting my writing. This book wouldn't have been possible without you. Your valuable feedback helps me grow as a writer. Oh, and thanks for those synonyms!

To my daughter, Shreya, and my sons, Shohan and Shomik: thank you for your positivity and encouragement. I'm so proud of each of you.

To my Ma: You're a gifted storyteller and an inspiration. I hope you enjoy reading this book and learning about iodine balance.

To my Baba: You left us too soon and I miss you every day. You were an incredible man and a wonderful father. I look to you for strength and guidance–always.

To my brother, Amit; sister, Mousumi; brother-in-law, Kingshuk; and sisters-in-law, Archana and Nandini: Thanks for always encouraging me and believing in my writing.

Thank you to my editors at Ulysses Press. You were a dream to work with, and I'm so grateful for your help and support during this writing journey.

About the Author

Malini Ghoshal, RPh, MS, is a published writer, speaker, and educator with a background in pharmacy. She has a master's in pharmaceutical policy and regulations. She writes for several major media organizations on a wide range of topics, including medications, health and wellness, mental health, health disparities, healthcare policy, and more. Her focus is on presenting well-researched, high-quality content that empowers individuals to lead healthier lives.

She is a passionate health advocate and has worked extensively with high-level federal, state, and community partners on major public health initiatives, including substance misuse prevention education.

Malini is strongly invested in improving health equity and outcomes for underrepresented groups. She has dedicated much of her health career to improving chronic disease health outcomes, both as a pharmacist and as a medical writer. More on her written work can be found at www.inspirra.com/healthcare.